MALPRACTICE

by JJ Perry

The contents of this work, including, but not limited to, the accuracy of events, people, and places depicted; opinions expressed; permission to use previously published materials included; and any advice given or actions advocated are solely the responsibility of the author, who assumes all liability for said work and indemnifies the publisher against any claims stemming from publication of the work.

All Rights Reserved
Copyright © 2019 by JJ Perry

No part of this book may be reproduced or transmitted, downloaded, distributed, reverse engineered, or stored in or introduced into any information storage and retrieval system, in any form or by any means, including photocopying and recording, whether electronic or mechanical, now known or hereinafter invented without permission in writing from the publisher.

Dorrance Publishing Co
585 Alpha Drive
Suite 103
Pittsburgh, PA 15238
Visit our website at *www.dorrancebookstore.com*

ISBN: 978-1-4809-8977-1
eISBN: 978-1-4809-9464-5

Chapter One

April 2004

Beads of sweat stuttered down Sarah's face as she leaned forward on the edge of her bed, gasping. 2:14 in large red numbers glared from the darkness into her panicked eyes. Her mouth gaped in rapid cadence, hungry for oxygen. Her lips pursed with each out-breath. Her cold, damp hands clutched her knees. Her arms trembled. Her feet chilled on the plush carpet.

As her breathing slowed she began to shiver. An ache gnawed in her belly, high under her ribs. She straightened to stretch it away. No help. She stood and the room tilted, turned. As soon as this stopped she shuffled into the bathroom and turned on the light. She clasped the heavy robe around her. In the mirror bloodshot eyes stared back at her from a deathly pale face. She moaned. *It's not a good day to be sick.*

A minute later her teeth chattered on her way back to bed. Lying flat, a smothering vice crushed her breath. She sat up and the constriction abated. She twisted the switch on a small, geometric bedside lamp and a low-wattage glow emerged. She pulled a couple of decorative stuffed shams together against the headboard, expedient but disorderly. She stopped for air. Over them she positioned her two down pillows in white Egyptian weave cases. Sitting with these propping her up, she initially puffed as if she had run a race but her breathing was better with her head up. She turned off the bedside lamp. Immediately fear thundered in and she turned it back on. She pulled the blanket and comforter high around her chin. Waves of trembling kept her wanting for comfort and rest that never fully came.

After four hours of restless dozing filled with dreadful dreams, she surrendered her hope for restful sleep. Finally warm, she rubbed her eyes and surveyed the room. No clothes on the floor, no clutter on the dressers met her gaze. There was no disorder anywhere except the bed. She flicked the radio alarm so it would not sound and got out of bed, dizzy again. She stood still as her vision tightened to a tunnel. She found herself on her knees, head on the bed almost in an attitude of prayer. She offered one quickly. Her vision brightened and her head stopped swimming. In caution, she stood. She carefully maneuvered to the master bath, feeling along the wall for balance. Her robe fell to the tile floor and she lifted her deep red negligee.

Standing up from the toilet, she observed the water, relieved to see no blood. Her abdominal discomfort had mostly eased, no longer alarming her. Her office opened in two hours but the tedious work she brought home demanded attention she could not give on a few hours fitful sleep. She had four days to complete a host of tax returns and corporate statements. In the mirror she pulled and fluffed the brown hair that had dried to her forehead. She tried to ignore the rest of the exhausted, bedraggled size 10 accountant whose face this time of year never yielded a sign of a spring tan. She turned away in frustration and eased into the hallway.

Amy, her nine-year-old daughter, slept undisturbed amidst a crowd of stuffed animals in the next room. Otherwise, the pleasant suburban home was empty, as it had been for seven years. She wanted to stroke Amy's chubby cheek as she often did but the short trip had already made her pant. She shuffled past into the kitchen to start coffee and lunches. She panted with pursed lips, gaining gradual relief.

She ground four level tablespoons of dark roasted beans exactly seventeen seconds and poured water into the spotless, stainless-steel drip coffeemaker to the precise mark of seven. When the gurgles told her the brew was in progress, piles of paper left from the night before beckoned from the third bedroom now turned office. Seven tax returns were neatly contained, each in a folder with the logo of Crawford & Benoit Accounting. Large manila envelopes hid the chaotic documentation from which order had been made. Stacks of protean notes were arranged around a partially completed 1040 form. Yellow Dixon Ticonderoga number-three lead pencils, razor sharp, lay perfectly aligned. Her writing, small, precise and left-leaning, revealed her personality. She knew that but couldn't change. She sighed at the unfinished projects and panted back to the kitchen, focused on making an egg salad sandwich using a hard-boiled egg pulled from a dimple in a tray on the refrigerator door without looking. Before she finished, she sat at the kitchen table, exhausted. Tax season was the worst possible time to be sick.

By the time she and Amy walked to the car inside the spotless garage, her breathing was easier. They didn't talk much, as usual. Amy's hair had been getting darker over the last year, no long pale blonde. Her round face with peculiar eyes characterized her Down syndrome. Usually Sarah tried to coax her to chat as they drove but not today. At Winkler, the special needs school, the short fourth grader loped off to join an array of other kids, many of them worse off than she.

Sarah then made the twenty-minute drive to near downtown Salt Lake City. She pulled into a parking garage and struggled with a bulging briefcase to reach her office inside the small firm with C & B logo and name painted on a glass door. She dropped her burden once inside, huffing with effort, face pale with strain. Her upper abdomen ached. Unnoticed so far, she hoisted her load and made it to her own small office and closed the door behind her. She took off her long wool coat and let it fall to the floor. It took her several minutes, to regain her wind but the night and morning convinced her to call her doctor. She pulled out a phone book in aggravation. The Yellow Pages tabbed "Physicians" were busy with colorful displays, like fishing lures. She found internal medicine and the name of her doctor. She sat in her ergonomic executive desk chair, left hand pressing her right lower ribcage while her other hand punched in the number.

"I need to see Dr. Barton today." Dolores Barton was part of a group of five internal medicine specialists located in a building attached to the Olympus Center of Healing Arts, a large urban hospital.

"She's not in today."

"I need to be seen. Should I go to the ER?"

"What is the problem?"

"My stomach hurts."

"If it's too painful, you should go to the emergency room or I can get another of our doctors see you about one o'clock this afternoon."

"This afternoon will be fine."

Sarah swallowed a couple of Tylenol and dug into the array of tax returns. She was irritated that she was sick enough to interrupt her work because each day before April 15th required as many hours as she could stay awake. The array of snapshots of Amy surrounding her office left her chronically guilty. She never spent enough time with her, especially during the three months of tax season.

Chapter Two

On the ground floor of the Marchetti building, a hospital completed in 1932 with classic granite and marble architecture, Don Zone presided over the Monday morning management meeting of Olympus Center of Healing Arts. In this office, the marble floor had been covered with thick wood underlayment, pad and carpet. Thin horizontal blinds modernized the windows while tropical plants, Euro-style furniture, a glass brick wall and a large Zen water feature added class. Jennifer Hayes, vice president and business director, had asked for questions following her presentation to the small group.

"So, when Saint Lucius Medical Center opens in July or so, they'll have trouble getting the big insurance players because of the way you wrote the contracts?" Zone asked.

"We gave them great rates if they gave us the right to refuse to add more hospitals to the network," responded Jennifer. She, pushing fifty years old and six feet in height, was bigger and older than her boss. "If they contract with Saint Lucius, the rates here go up thirty-five percent. Since we provide the majority of care in the valley, I doubt they'll allow their insureds to use the new hospital."

"That'll make Saint's startup very expensive." Don glowed, a short forty-seven-year-old triathlete. "Perfect!"

"I had another idea that might really bury them," Jennifer said as she flicked lint off her tan lapel. She had a penchant for blazers with the somewhat dominating masculine look and an ability to hide about twenty pounds. "Are you ready for this?"

The two men nodded.

"One of Saint's goals is to compete with our cardiovascular service line. They made an attractive offer to Chandler Cardiovascular to relocate their office from here to there."

"We can't let that happen," Zone said. He was master of the obvious, she often quipped, a stupid jock that she led around by the nose. The men or, as she usually said, the boys, at the corporate headquarters in Houston, preferred athletic or alcoholic men over more competent women and she tired of it. Maybe this time, she could prove her worth.

"Malouf, their new leader, is financially driven. I have a way of beating Saint's offer: keeping the group here and essentially boycotting their programs."

"Corporate's been in trouble with physician arrangements in the past," said Chad Mixon, the chief financial officer, six and a half feet tall, skinny and gray at age forty-two.

Auspicious HealthCare owned Olympus and about forty other hospitals in the country. Jennifer was politicking for a job at their office in Houston.

"I started brainstorming with Malouf three or four months ago," she said. "We provide them with a cardiac cath lab."

"I thought we were going to add a fourth lab here," Chad said.

"That was the plan. We need more capacity. But Chandler owns the lab that creates incentive to keep all their outpatient work here."

"That'll cost us a lot more money both to buy it and the lost revenue," Chad whined. "Not nearly as much as we'll lose if they start a competing heart surgery program."

"There's a law against us providing physicians with that sort of incentive. Auspicious will never approve," Chad said.

"The money will be channeled in such a way that we're safe from discovery."

"Should I ask how? That sounds illegal."

"I wouldn't use that term," Don chastised. "What I want from you, Chad, is to run the numbers."

"Got it." He nodded his acquiescence.

"I have a meeting with Malouf for lunch today," Hayes said. "I'd like to tell her we're moving ahead with corporate approval and the legal work."

"Good idea," Zone said. "Make it happen. Between blocking their insurance contracts and killing the cardiovascular program, Saints will fold within a year or two. I love eating not-for-profits." He stood, stretching his legs and arms.

Hayes knew what he was thinking when his jaw muscles flexed and relaxed. *He wanted to get to the gym for a couple of hours to feed his competitive hunger. Good, because everyone was better off with him out of the building.*

CHAPTER 3

Most of the year there were frequent interruptions for Sarah by other accountants or clerks wanting to talk. No such chatter this day would have allowed her to move through her work efficiently. Her vague discomfort distracted her, robbed her appetite and kept her looking at the clock as if relief would come from the approaching appointment. She left the building twenty minutes before one, carrying papers for a few returns she could prepare as she waited.

Wasatch Creeks Medical Associates was a well-run practice. Within ten minutes of arrival, Sarah was in a paper gown, seated on an exam table freezing and shivering. Her toes and fingers were blue. She put her coat over her gown after less than a minute of waiting. A medical assistant came in, a youngish plump woman who was pierced and chatty. She took her temperature: 98.1, her pulse: 105, and her blood pressure: 92/54. The young woman noted her discomfort and fetched a warm blanket.

A few minutes later a short, trim, young-looking man in a brown shirt and blue tie walked in, a stethoscope draped around his neck and a chart in his hands. His haircut was short, tight, obsessive. He offered his skinny, limp hand. "I'm Doctor Wren. How can I help you today?" He had coffee breath and cold fingers.

"My stomach hurts," she said, placing her right hand over the edge of her ribs at the top of her abdomen. "It woke me up about two in the morning. I had a hard time breathing."

"Does it hurt bad?"

"I wouldn't be here if it wasn't keeping me from working."

"Does it radiate anywhere from the right side? Into your back or chest?"

"No."

"Short of breath, you said?"

"Yes."

"Does it hurt to breathe in deep?"

"Not much. Maybe a little. I can't tell." She inhaled, feeling for a change.

He asked more questions and perused her record, struggling to read the penmanship in places. She thought things would have run faster with Dr. Barton since she had an uncomplicated medical history other than a remote year of ulcerative colitis and took no medications except occasional antihistamines, cough syrup and an inhaler. Her prior laboratory studies had been normal. Importantly, her chart was thin, a sign of good health like a thin envelope usually meant a simple tax return.

Wren sent her to the hospital through a sconce-lighted corridor to X-ray and the clinical lab. She was convinced that this was overkill, that she didn't have time for a bunch of tests, that she was healthy with some sort of virus or something that would go away as quickly as it came. She thought about just going back to work but she had to slow down twice on the walk to catch her breath.

Afterward, a thin blonde woman pushed her back to the office in a wheelchair. Sarah thanked her. The orderly made a quiet comment to an older nurse. Sarah returned to her room where she opened a tax return. She had just started when the same medical assistant returned and had her lie on the exam table for a few minutes. She then repeated her blood pressure lying, sitting and standing, making notes.

With a couple of sheets of paper in hand, Wallace Wren returned. Sarah put down her pencil and calculator, wiped hair back from her eyes and waited for him to speak.

"Your chest X-ray is not normal. It's hard to say if you have pneumonia or perhaps a blood clot. Your heart is generous, borderline enlarged. Your bloodwork shows a high white blood cell count and slightly elevated enzymes. Your blood pressure is low. Maybe that is how you are but it is lower than it was on your previous visits and it falls when you stand up."

Sarah said nothing as he continued his presentation.

"Bottom line, you need to be in the hospital at least overnight so we can do more tests. This could be something serious." He stopped talking.

"Could it wait two or three days?"

"No. If it's a blood clot in your lung you could be dead before morning." He frowned.

She put her face in both hands and shook her head, as if trying to wake up from a nightmare.

"Your symptoms and lab values indicate you need to be hospitalized. We'll find the diagnosis faster as we keep an eye on you." He ran a hand over his cropped hair.

"My daughter has Down syndrome and I'm a single parent. I'll need to make some arrangements for her."

"You'll have time to make some calls."

"I just can't do this now. I'm up to my neck in tax returns with three days to finish."

"I don't know that your condition is life threatening but it could be. It would be malpractice not to put you in the hospital."

She grimaced in pain and frustration. "This is horrible."

"Let me walk you to the nursing desk and see if we were able to get you a room."

Sarah stood up and collected her things as Dr. Wren stepped outside the doorway. As she hefted the satchel strap to her shoulder she felt dizzy and the room began to dim. She saw the floor come quickly to her face. Extending an arm, she broke her fall. Papers scattered everywhere. A rushing sound filled her ears mixed with voices not making sense. She willed herself to see, hear and think but it was slow to happen.

"Get a gurney! She has a pulse. She's breathing! See if the blood pressure cuff will stretch down here. Sarah, are you okay?"

"I'll be fine," she willed in the flurry of activity surrounding her.

Dr. Wren looked down at her, his face filled with concern.

CHAPTER 4

Chandler Cardiovascular Clinic was named after Randolph Betts Chandler, a cardiologist who began a solo consulting practice thirty years earlier, merged with Hugh Harrison and Nigel Sampson, and died a few years later, leaving Hugh to manage the practice. Rather than call themselves *Cardiovascular Con-*

sultants like almost every other group in the country, they kept Chandler's name. The Clinic had grown to a dozen cardiologists, half a dozen nurse practitioners or physician's assistants and about seventy other employees. The clinic occupied one floor of the four-story office building attached to OCHA by a bridge about one hundred fifty feet long above a busy avenue. They had smaller offices in nearby towns, Park City and Layton.

At the end of the day, after office patients had left, three doctors sat at one end of a long table in their boardroom.

"What did Gullimore say?" Stanton Bleeker Blackstone was forty plus, six feet tall, about two hundred thirty pounds and a perpetual five o'clock shadow. He had been a full partner in the practice for six years and looked forward to the top seat, now occupied by a woman: Sarisha Malouf.

"He says the contract does not say what we all thought it said. We should just let Harrison leave in August as he planned. We won't need to pay him more than $12,000." Malouf smiled as she spoke, her dark eyes exuding triumph and revenge. She was the current chief executive of the practice, a cardiologist whose specialty was echocardiography and other non-invasive cardiac imaging.

"You're kidding," responded Blackstone with thick raised eyebrows. "That sounds a lot better than eight hundred thousand. How come?" He wanted her job that she had held over a year. His bid failed then. She achieved it by seniority, not merit, Blackstone had often grumbled.

"I told you Gullimore was a good attorney. He said we won't need to pay Harrison his deferred compensation or his accounts receivable. I was afraid we would also need to buy back his stock at market value. He said we don't, as long as he works in Salt Lake, or anywhere in this county. He loses everything except the stock. It's all in the non-compete clause."

"The stock that we intentionally undervalued when he gave notice," Blackstone said.

"I thought neither he nor Sampson had a non-compete," Montgomery Pierce said.

"Well, they do, according to Gullimore," she said. "And that changes everything. We won't have to come up with a huge sum in the fall."

"Bonuses intact!" Blackstone said. "Hallelujah." He didn't like working under a woman boss but it was better than the atheist tyrant Harrison. Malouf and Pierce were also a lot better with money. His income was rising a lot with her running the show.

"I'll have Gullimore come to our monthly meeting a week from Monday, when Harrison is away."

"I am so tired of covering for his research junkets," Blackstone moaned.

"You're on call that weekend anyway, Stan," Malouf said. "Man up."

"He's the sucker willing to bring studies here," Pierce said. "It makes us look good and breaks even financially."

"We make a little," Malouf agreed without enthusiasm.

"Whatever," Blackstone said. "I have to run. See you tomorrow." His watch said a quarter before six as he rode the elevator to his new black Infiniti parked under the clinic. Bible school started at six-thirty. He had to first pick up Stacey, his wife, and their one-year-old daughter, Rachel, which meant he had to hurry.

Blackstone gritted his teeth as he revved the turbo engine and screeched out of the lot. Harrison had hired him ten years ago, fresh out of training. He felt a twinge of conscience about disliking him so intensely. It was not Christian. *"Love thine enemies. Do good for those that spitefully use you."* He knew he had been used, worked like a rented mule, then disrespected just for a few complications that weren't his fault. For years Harrison had flitted around the country while he stayed in town, keeping one end of the practice running, seeing scores of patients and doing more work than almost any of the other cardiologists. Part of him wanted to stop hating this godless and immoral partner for it might canker his soul. He prayed briefly as he eased his dry and shiny car through other cars beaded with the slush of new April snow.

"He's impetuous," Pierce said after Blackstone left. "That comes in handy at times."

"I always wonder what you are thinking, Monty," she said.

"Just ways of bringing more success to our endeavor."

He said success. She heard money.

"Gin and tonic?" he asked.

Loose-jowled and mostly gray, he looked trustworthy. She nodded. She didn't trust him at all.

She was in her mid-forties and had been through residency twice like a lot of foreign physicians, once in Lebanon and again in Houston. Right after cardiology training, Dr. Chandler offered her a job, which she declined. She joined later, after the merger and two weeks before he had failed to show up for work because he was dead in a recliner in front of his television; kindly killed by the disease he treated. Had she taken his initial offer, she would have had the corner office. It had taken years to claim the control she deserved and coveted.

She turned her attention to the letter from Jon Gullimore, attorney at law, which contained an analysis of the employment contract Harrison and all shareholding cardiologists had signed. She and Pierce reread the language.

"The meaning depends on what word you emphasize," she said.

"The moron we hired to write this a few years ago made it deliciously ambiguous," Pierce said. "Legal malpractice, but it'll work well for us."

"Harrison will fight this," she said.

"Considering his enormous alimony, I doubt he has the resources. There are a dozen of us to fund a war. He cannot possible win."

Malouf glowed in schadenfreude. "Then I hope he goes deep into debt just to lose."

"That's the spirit," Pierce said, lifting his glass of Scotch. She clinked it with her gin and tonic.

If her guess were anywhere near correct, the fifty-year-old would be left with nothing but inflated alimony payments, which came courtesy of a Utah tradition. She believed that Harrison's managerial incompetence had resulted in a forty-percent drop in the income of every clinic doctor for two years. She wanted him to suffer. In reality, the reduction in pay happened after Pierce had managed for a year, bungled the finances and acquired significant debt.

Chapter 5

Sarah lay in room 3433 feeling fine. It was a fresh room, newly carpeted, wallpapered and wood paneled on an internal medicine ward of Hunter Tower. Bleached white sheets and a woven cotton blanket lay over legs pulled up to her abdomen. The window looked over a parking lot, a maintenance building and homes. Not far away were snowcapped mountains, not visible in the twilight and slushy rain. April was always wet. She lifted up the phone and redialed her ex-husband yet again. After four rings she was about to hang up when he answered.

"Doug, this is Sarah. Did you pick up Amy?"

"Yeah. She's here. We went to McDonald's for dinner."

"I was worried when no one answered at your home."

"Sorry. Can't afford a cell phone, as you know."

"Couldn't use a few bucks of the alimony I pay you and get something basic?" She could never resist making the same jab about money.

"Two beers a day is more important than a phone," he countered.

"How's Amy?"

"She's fine."

"Can I talk to her?"

"Just a minute."

Amy could not be far away. He lived in a one-bedroom apartment, maybe five or six hundred square feet, old and cheap. She heard rustling. "Hello?"

"Hi, Amy! This is Mom."

"Daddy says you're sick."

"I'm afraid so, honey. The doctor won't let me come home until I'm better."

"I want to see you."

"It's late tonight. I'll ask Daddy if he'll bring you over after school. Is that okay?"

"I want you come home."

"I'll be there in a day or two."

Amy began to cry.

Doug took the phone and said, "She's upset."

Sarah swallowed her usual insult, *master of the obvious,* and exhaled to regain her calm.

"Would you bring her to see me at the hospital tomorrow after school? It'd help her to see me."

"Won't you be home?"

"I don't know. If I'm not, she needs to see me."

"It's going to be inconvenient."

"It's for your daughter's sake."

"Will you pay for the gas?"

"Have you no shame?"

"None." He spoke with a matter-of-fact air.

"You live maybe four miles away and get over twenty miles a gallon in that old Datsun.

So, less than half a gallon of gas. I'll give you a dollar."

"We'll be over then."

"Do you have her medicine for tonight and in the morning?"

"What medicine?"

"The pink bottle I told you about."

"Oh, that. Don't have it. She forgot."

"She's the one with—" Sarah choked back another insult. "She needs the medicine for three more days. It's an antibiotic. Could you please go get it?"

"I don't know." He laughed.

Sarah hung up. She wiped sweat from her brow. Doug had been a charming bad boy, a refreshing change from a boring, compulsive accountant boyfriend she had dated for a couple of years. She soon became pregnant, married him and quickly found his charm was a facade. She divorced him within two years.

There was a knock on the door as Dr. Wren entered. His blue tie was askew; he looked haggard at the end of his thirteen-hour day. "Hi, Mrs. Thompson. How are you?"

"It's no worse."

"You look a little winded. Do you feel short of breath?"

"No. I'm just sitting here in bed." She realized she was breathing a little faster than usual and attributed it to irritation with Doug. "What about my tests?"

"That's why I'm here. Your CT scan did not show any blood clots in your lungs. That's good. Your repeat bloodwork still shows some mildly elevated liver enzymes and white count. Your temperature is up and your blood pressure down. We have some cultures cooking that should show some results tomorrow. I've ordered some different enzymes and blood tests for the morning."

"What are you thinking, Dr. Wren?"

"Maybe you have hepatitis, though I doubt it. You might have an infection but your urine looks pretty clean other than a little protein. There's no pneumonia. If you're not doing better tomorrow and if things are still unclear, I might have a specialist or two take a look at you."

"Do you think I'll go home tomorrow?"

"Let's discuss that in the morning."

At 4:15 Tuesday morning a strand of muscle fibers of Sarah's Thompson's heart fired on its own, well before the signal of a normal beat would arrive. This is a normal and common occurrence, a premature ventricular contraction or PVC. But in her case, the electrical process also found a circuitous pathway of muscle cells that were slow to fire causing a dozen beats at a rate around two hundred per minute before it stopped. Had this occurred to her on a cardiac ward, alarms would have sounded and a nurse would have hurried in to check on her. However, Sarah was on a medical floor where her heart rhythm was not monitored. No one saw this pre-lethal rhythm, ventricular tachycardia or VT, despite occurring half a dozen times in the predawn hours. It woke her up a couple of times, though she no idea why.

Before 6:00 a thin, young woman with hair dyed coal black and lipstick only slightly lighter entered Sarah's room, tightened a bright blue elastic around her upper arm and withdrew four more small vials of blood, hardly disturbing her sleep. In a tube with a red and black "tiger" top, the blood clotted within minutes. Half an hour later that tube was in a centrifuge that separated the semisolid coagulum from yellow serum. Ten minutes later, a technician pipetted her serum into a small vial, which was placed into a large analyzer. About an hour after the blood was drawn, a sheet flew out of a laser printer on Three East Tower, a medical unit. It was the change of shift, a noisy, bustling, daily confusion. It was one piece of paper among of scores of similar reports. A yawning clerk, out late the night before collected the lab sheets and distributed them into charts between strokes of her long, straight streaked hair.

By 7:45, the night shift nurses were mostly gone. Sarah stood up from her bed with a nurse's aide at her side. Once again she felt lightheaded. She put an arm out as she started to fall. The sturdy young woman held her up.

Dr. Wren walked into Sarah's room at that moment. "What's going on?" he asked and hurried over to help get Sarah back into bed.

"I got dizzy when I got up to go to the bathroom," she managed after lying down.

Wren checked her pulse. It was one hundred thirty. "Take her blood pressure, please," he directed the young aide.

She returned quickly with a wheeled tower with a vital sign machine attached. Wren asked questions. "Did you feel okay until you got up?"

"Yes."

"Have you had any chest pain?"

"No. My stomach still hurts about the same."

"Have you been short of breath?"

"Not really."

"I have to transfer you to the telemetry floor. Your blood test from this morning showed an elevation of a cardiac enzyme. We need to monitor your rhythm. I'm also ordering an echocardiogram and an EKG."

"What does that mean?"

"I still don't know what's going on but with elevated enzymes, we need to look at your heart."

"It's my stomach that hurts."

"Your blood tells a different story. So, you've had no discomfort in your chest?"

"No. Well, I mean I woke up a few times with a strange feeling." She placed her hand at the top of her breastbone and sighed. "My clients are going to kill me if I don't get their taxes done."

He glanced at the blood pressure reading that just popped up on the mobile cart. "You need to stay here for at least another day. Your blood pressure falls when you stand up and it's low already."

"This is the worst possible time."

"Let's check your pressure when you're standing."

He and the aide helped Sarah out of bed. Wren held on to her as she began to sway as the aide punched the blood pressure button. Sarah began to crumple but they managed to get her on to the bed. The screen on the machine indicated her pressure was not obtainable

"Are you okay?" Dr. Wren asked.

"Really lightheaded," she gasped.

"You're okay staying in the hospital?"

"Yeah."

He left the room and wrote orders the transfer, an echocardiogram and a cardiology consult from Hugh Harrison, the leader of Chandler Cardiovascular and, in Wren's opinion, the best cardiologist in the state.

By early afternoon Sarah was in room 4315, part of the Cardiac Treatment Unit, CTU, also known as Four North Tower. Her heart's electrical signal was now continuously displayed and monitored on a bank of screens. Dr. Dolores Barton encountered a short, happy echocardiographic technician wheeled her large machine down the hall away from Sarah's room.

"Did you do the echo on Thompson?" Barton asked. "Just finished."

"What did you find?"

The technician hesitated. Barton knew the rules, that the techs were not to report on the echoes. "Just what you think. I won't tell."

"Her valves are okay. Her ejection fraction is a little low." The ejection fraction referred to a measure of the strength and function of the heart. A normal ventricle squeezes out 50 to 70 percent of its blood volume with each heartbeat. In a weak ventricle, or pumping chamber, the fraction of blood ejected falls.

"What was her E. F.?"

"I got 45 percent."

"Humph." She wrinkled her brow as she walked away too concerned to offer any thanks.

"Has Harrison been in to see fifteen yet?" She asked the ward clerk, to whom room numbers supplanted names.

"I haven't seen him."

She sat next to the monitor tech, nudging her over a bit so she could sit in front of the bank of heart monitors. She clicked on Sarah's rectangle and reviewed her rhythm. It showed one four beat run of VT but otherwise had been normal although her rate was still a little fast, about one hundred ten beats per minute.

The monitor tech stood and gave her chair to Theodore W. Hatcher, a cardiologist, who joined Dolores at the monitors. "Hi, Ted," she said.

He looked at the display of VT. "Need a cardiologist?"

"I called Harrison," she said.

"You knew he's leaving, right?"

"I knew he was leaving Chandler. When is that?"

"Not soon enough." Her face made it clear the answer was inadequate. "August," he grumbled.

"Why did you guys force him out? He's the kingpin."

"I think he's burned out. After he was voted out of leadership, he probably couldn't stand to see anyone else, especially Sarisha, running the place." Ted turned to face her more directly, his eyes running up and down, side to side.

Dolores assumed he liked what he saw, as did many men. Early forties, tall, brunette, Teutonic bones and face, body fit, muscular. She made some effort to keep her ample chest well hidden, seldom using that asset, at least overtly, to gain advantage. He ran his hand through his long dark hair.

"It's hard to fathom that he would voluntarily leave the group he built," she said.

To most people in the local medical community it was known as Harrison's group, not Chandler. The difference in the two men was great. Chandler attracted referrals from doctors due to his magnetic self-confidence and aggressive approach to problems. Harrison was a self-deprecating leader. He didn't always agree with her about doing procedures she wanted done but when he got into the cath lab, he was legendary. He had bailed out many of his partners from some crisis or another but they still wanted him out.

"You men and your petty politics," she said.

"I think the clinic will be better off without him." He shrugged.

Another string of four rapid, fat blips slid smoothly across the screen and disappeared within six seconds. Her eyebrow moved up as Hatcher droned on. An alarm sounded softly and a strip of skinny paper peeled out with the four beats printed, all without human interaction.

"I can't believe he is joining the idiots at the International Chest Institute."

"Really? That gang of below average docs with such a grandiose title," Dolores responded, although she wanted to offer her overused joke that it was the clinic named after her dominant anatomic characteristic. "Those guys have fought for years."

"He'll tear that group apart, drive them into ruin."

Maybe he'll turn that group into the premier cardiology practice as he had Chandler Cardiovascular, she thought. She ripped the piece of ECG paper off the machine and walked back to her chart. "Got to keep moving. Lunch break is almost over."

After half a dozen steps she glanced back. Hatcher had been watching her, her tight black slacks, her stair-stepper butt. She winked. He looked away.

As she neared room 4315, staccato heel clicks dotted the silence. When she got to the doorway, she found scraps of paper spilling out of a manila envelope, assorted in shape, size and color. Sarah looked up.

"You're back," Sarah remarked.

"Yes, and I didn't expect to find you here. It doesn't look like you're resting."

Stacks of folders lay on a counter on the side of the room, tax forms and papers lay in a distinct orthogonal pattern on the bedside table and the bed.

"People depend on me to get this done."

"How are you feeling?"

"I feel better, actually." She forced a smile. "My stomach seems almost back to normal." "Have you been out of bed much?"

"Just to the bathroom. Other than this morning, that seems fine. I just had a heart test. Did it show anything?"

"A cardiologist needs to read it before we know anything. How's your daughter?"

"Amy is fine, thanks."

Dr. Barton quickly examined Sarah, listened carefully to her lungs and heart, poked in her belly and legs as they talked. She stood straight and draped her stethoscope around her neck then tugged on her tan corduroy vest. "You look good to me. But your heart rhythm has been a little unsteady. I'll be interested to hear what Dr. Harrison thinks when he sees you later. I hope we can get you home tomorrow."

"Tonight would be better."

"We'll see." This always meant no.

When Barton got back to the charting area, Hatcher was gone, thankfully.

Chapter 6

"I'm Dr. Harrison. Dr. Barton asked if I would see you."

His oily, dark hair rimmed a pate where few strands grew long and rebellious. Unruly sideburns emerged below that but the most glaring out of style feature was his pencil thin mustache. His droopy facial folds gave an impression of excesses and deficiencies.

"I'm the cardiologist."

Outside, the dinner trays rattled as they were wheeled onto the Cardiac Treatment Unit.

"Oh, yeah. Okay." She sat up straight and cross-legged under the light blue blanket. She fluffed her hospital gown in front of her, trying to relieve the tension that had hit at the sound of his specialty.

"Is this a good time to visit?"

"Of course. I want to go home today. As soon as I am through seeing you and the gastroenterologist, I hope to leave." She lifted her papers to show that she was busy, had deadlines, could not possible stay one hour longer.

"Have you ever had heart trouble?"

"No"

"Have you had chest pain?" The questions were many. He wanted to know if she had been short of breath, had swollen ankles, had palpitations, high blood pressure and on. What were her habits, her diet; how about her family? His interview style was efficient and professional, devoid of judgment. Other than her current problem he found she had been healthy except for about a year of colitis when her marriage disintegrated.

He studied her neck, touching it lightly, then pushed below her ribs. "What are you doing?"

"I'm checking your neck veins. They're a little plump."

"Plump?"

"You have too much fluid."

"You can tell that by just looking?"

"Your veins are like a dipstick." He smiled.

She smiled back. He was funny in a dry way.

He listened to her chest front and back, prodded her belly again, probed her shins and stood back. "You have a gallop. Your liver is a little big. Your veins are distended. You have what we call heart failure."

"Dr. Barton said nothing about that."

"I looked at your echo before coming to see you," he continued. "Your left ventricle, the main pumping chamber, is normal in size but looks a little sluggish. When that is combined with a small elevation in cardiac muscle enzyme, it means an injury to your heart. If you were older, I'd think heart attack. However, combined with some things I found on your examination it's something else. It would be unwise to let you go home now, especially because your heart rhythm is occasionally erratic."

She wanted to scream. An older woman wearing a black apron and pants, white shirt and goofy cravat entered carrying a tray of dinner. Sarah moved her tax returns off the bedside table to make room for the questionable smelling food.

"Here you go, girl. Enjoy!" she bustled out.

"Thank you!" Sarah called out.

"We'll do more blood tests and another heart test tomorrow," Harrison said. "I'm going to start you on some medication that I think will speed up your recovery. Most people just get better without treatment but we don't know that will be the case with you."

Sarah avoided eye contact in her disappointment. "How long will I be in here?"

"It's hard to say without seeing how you do. At least two more days, I would guess." "What kind of a test will I have?"

"It will involve drawing some blood, attaching a little bit of radioactive material to the cells, then reinjecting it. This is a very accurate way of measuring your heart function, more reproducible than the echo. We call it a MUGA scan."

He waited for her to ask another question. None came.

"I'm sure you're scared or nervous. Chances are good that you'll get over this quickly. Anything else you want to know?"

"I don't know enough to ask questions." While she had many physician clients, she knew nothing about medicine except the finances.

"I'll check on you in the morning." He left.

She looked at the pile of work and shook her head. She couldn't do all that was needed from a hospital bed. She had done enough on these returns to determine an approximate payment, if any, to submit with the extension. It was time to plan the retreat. She called one of her colleagues and asked him to pick up her unfinished work tomorrow and file for extensions where needed.

As Harrison left noticed a wiry tanned and tattooed man towed a resistant and unhappy dark blonde girl with the characteristic appearance of Down syndrome toward the nursing station.

"Are you here to see Sarah?" he asked.

"Mommy," Amy said.

The man just nodded. Harrison pointed to room fifteen.

Sarah looked up from her watery potatoes, red goulash and soggy green beans to see Amy enter. Her frown fractured into a broad small-toothed smile as she pounced on her mother. Sarah wrapped her up and hugged until she couldn't breathe. They went forehead to forehead and looked at each other out of focus. Noses rubbed and giggles blurped. Separating a little, Sarah tenderly coddled the face of her girl, stoking her cheek with a thumb, fingers massaging the back of her neck.

"Amy, I'm so glad you came." She pushed the dinner tray away.

"Daddy brought me."

"Did you miss me?"

"A bunch. This much!" She stretched her hands as far apart as possible to demonstrate. "More than that even," she added.

"I missed you twice that," Sarah said.

"I missed you the mostest," Amy said.

"I wish so much I could be home," she said. "My doctors said it would be a few more days."

"You don't look sick," Doug said.

Amy turned and responded to her father's skepticism. "Mommy's sick inside." She looked back at Sarah. "Right, Mommy?"

"That's right, sweetie." She caressed her daughter's small, round head, kissing her with her gaze. "In here." She put her other hand on her solar plexus and patted.

"I'd like to talk to your doctor," Doug said.

"We are not related, Doug. Just butt out."

"Have you called Myra and Ed?" Her parents.

"Of course."

Amy picked up a white plastic box with a long cord, turning it over in her miniature hands. "What's this?"

"Don't interrupt, Amy. Adults are having a conversation."

"Doug, it's okay. She's just curious."

"She needs to learn manners."

"Like you could teach her?"

"Insult me more and you'll need to find another way to get Amy home."

"You'd abandon your child just to make a point?"

He glowered.

Sarah noticed that Amy had hit the call button. Amy's face showed the dismay that always appeared in conflict.

A male nurse with light hair, faded freckles, one earring and light blue scrubs came in, "Aaron" on his ID. "Do you need something?"

"Could you show this man to the waiting room?"

"I need to watch over my daughter. She's retarded."

"I'm sure she'll be fine here, Sir. The waiting room is just—"

"I know where the goddam waiting room is, faggot." Doug shook his shoulder-length hair and looked down at the kid, about four inches shorter than his almost six foot height.

"Daddy!" Amy did her best attempt to scowl at him.

"Do you have to pick a fight everywhere you go?" Sarah said.

"Are you related?" Aaron asked.

"Divorced a long time ago," Sarah said.

"Wish you had a hot nurse instead of a homo."

"I'm so sorry," Sarah said. "Doug, please. Give Amy and me a few minutes."

"Do I need to call security?" Aaron asked.

"You don't need to call anybody. I'm protecting my daughter." He put a hand under his long-tailed, unbuttoned and untucked shirt, as if reaching for something tucked in his belt. He stared as the young man backed into the hallway and away from the room.

Unaware of what was happening in room fifteen, Dr. Harrison had walked off the ward to see two more patients needing Friday evening consultation. Behind him a musical alarm went off at the telemetry station as a strip of paper from Sarah's monitor coiled on the desk, showing the longest run of ventricular tachycardia of the day.

"Looks like you have been working," Doug said, pointing at the stacks of returns.

"So I can pay your damn alimony."

"God bless America."

"Are you out of work again?"

"Ski season is over, so yeah. Life is good."

"Do you want to hear about school today, Mommy?"

"I do. What did you learn today?"

As they talked, Sarah touched her daughter often.

Aaron called security. A pair of overweight men in blue shirts and mesh vests exited the elevator a couple of minutes later.

"So, is he armed?" one of them asked.

"I didn't see a weapon," Aaron replied. "But he reached for something under his shirt."

The pair looked at each other. They could have been forty years apart.

"Well, I'll talk to him," said the older man. "You stay back a little."

"Sir," he called out at the threshold of room fifteen. "May I have a word with you?"

Sarah looked at the security guard blocking the door and hugged Amy close. Doug was resting on one foot, the other leg crossed over, shoulder pressed on the wall.

He turned to face the man. "What do you want, skipper?"

"Step out into the hall so we can speak, please."

"I don't think so. This woman might molest my child."

"How about if my associate keeps an eye on things in here while we talk?" Sweat beaded and rolled down the plethoric face of the pudgy junior guard.

"Nah." He turned to watch Sarah and Amy.

The senior guard thought for a moment. "Ma'am, would you like this man to stay in your room?"

Sarah weighed the alternatives and the projected consequences before she answered. "I'd like him out."

Doug shrugged off the wall and stepped deeper into the room, sitting on the foot of the bed, facing the door, right hand resting at his belt under his shirt, out of sight.

"Doug," she said calmly, "get off my bed and out of the room."

"Not without Amy."

"We're not through visiting."

"Well, then, finish up. My bitch is waiting."

"Sir, please step outside. I just need a word with you, that's all. It doesn't need to be complicated."

"Let's get out of here," he said to Amy, clinging to her mom with all her strength. "Let's go."

He reached out both arms toward her. She didn't move.

"Amy, maybe it's better if you go. We can visit tomorrow. I'll have Grandma bring you and you can stay as long as you like, honey."

The silence was broken by a distant voice of an elderly woman repeatedly calling, "Nurse, nurse, nurse!"

Amy kissed Sarah hard on the lips, tears in her eyes. "Bye, bye, Mommy." She slid off the bed on the opposite side of Doug and walked toward the guard.

Doug met her at the foot, picked up her hand and held it. She did not squeeze back.

As Doug walked past the old guard, he defiantly swung his shoulder at him, missing by a fraction of an inch. Amy looked back as they left until the image of her mother disappeared around the frame. They moved slowly toward the elevator, Doug keeping his right hand under his shirttail all the while. Peaches followed at a distance.

"Is that your husband?" the older guy asked from the threshold.

"Not for years," she answered.

"Does he have a record? He seems mean."

"I wouldn't be surprised. He's angry all the time."

"Has he beat you up?"

"Not since the divorce."

"What's his name? I'm going to have the police keep an eye on him. I think we'll also want to stay close if he comes back to visit."

At the elevator, a man with a cane limped off as Doug and Amy got in. He lugged a large satchel that hunched his back and lengthen his jowls. He studied the signs before heading into CTU, toward room fifteen. Full head of brown hair, graying at the temples, in need of a trim framed a sallow face. Soft hands extended from his well-worn tweed jacket with corduroy at the elbows. When he got to the door, Sarah had her face in both hands.

"Is everything okay, Sarah?"

She looked up. "Hi, Bill. My ex was just here doing what he does best, that's all."

"How are you doing?" He looked concerned.

"I didn't need you to come tonight. I can finish a couple more of these before morning. I just... I don't think I can finish all these and get them back to the clients for signature by tomorrow night."

"You're being ridiculous. You're in the hospital for a reason and need to rest. I'm taking everything with me."

"I have finished all but these returns." She pointed at a stack. "And for them I have estimated taxes due for the filing." She went through the details carefully handwritten in tiny, neat letters on two legal-sized yellow papers.

He left five minutes later, leaving her without a single piece of paper. She put her head back on the pillow and let tears flow.

Chapter 6

Saturday, April 15, debuted at midnight with Harrison in the cardiac catheterization laboratory treating an eighty-seven-year-old woman with a heart attack.

Later, when the sun was well up, Dr. Barton entered Sarah's room, greeted by the familiar odor of vomit. With her face down, Sarah's eyes moved from the off-pink plastic basin to the visitor. Barton noted sweat dripping from her hair and nose. She saw Sarah's bed was cranked to an upright position, that her arms trembled, barely balancing the bucket on her lap. Moving closer, she saw green, watery fluid with a few clumps of partially digested dinner. Sarah's head flopped back onto the pillow in exhaustion. Her skin seemed translucent. Perspiration soaked her cotton gown about four inches down from the neck.

"Hi," Sarah croaked.

"When did you start throwing up?"

"A few minutes ago."

An aide bustled into the room, pushing the button that cancelled the call light. She quickly helped with the container and wiped Sarah's face with a white washcloth, then stroked her back in a comforting gesture.

"How was your night?"

"Those night nurses know how to party." She attempted a smile.

"Would you check her vitals?" Barton asked the aide, who then left in search of a machine.

She felt for the pulse in Sarah's wrist. It took a while to find it, small, weak and rapid, about 120 per minute. She counted breaths. Six in fifteen seconds, twenty-four a minute was high but not serious. "Would it be okay if I lowered the head of your bed?"

"Yeah."

The angle decreased. When it got to about thirty degrees, Sarah tried to lift a hand. "That's enough. Thanks." Her voice was barely audible, mostly a whisper.

Barton felt her forehead. Cold. Placing a stethoscope on her back, the expanding lungs sounded clear. She looked for distended neck veins and saw some wiggles under her ear, probably what Harrison had seen. She listened and heard the extra sound of a stressed heart, the "gallop" he reported.

"Are you feeling a little better now?"

"A little bit, yeah."

The aide rolled in a pole with the vital sign machine attached.

"It looks like Dr. Harrison ordered a different scan for today. Otherwise, we have nothing planned. Just waiting for you to get better."

"Just tell me what to do."

"You just need to rest. Can I do something for you now?"

"No.

"Did you see your little girl last night?"

"It was a short visit," she croaked wistfully.

"I'm on call for the weekend so I'll be in tomorrow. See you then, Sarah."

"Thank you, Dr. Barton." She managed a partial smile for Dolores as she left.

She found Hugh Harrison bent over the bank of heart monitors in the nursing station and said, "Hey."

"Thanks for letting me see your patient," Harrison said. "What do you think is going on with her?"

"Probably acute myocarditis." Med-speak for a Myocardial Infarction or heart attack. "I should probably do an angiogram to make certain it's not an occluded vessel."

"She's too young for a heart attack."

"I've seen younger. Her enzyme level fell this morning so that's good. As long as she is stable, I'll probably wait until Monday. It'll give her a chance to get used to the idea."

"What's this with leaving Chandler?"

"The inmates took over the asylum."

She said nothing in response.

"The new hires are in control. They vote on doing things that I just can't live with."

"Like what?"

"All sorts of things. The group values have changed since we became big. And they're working on a deal with the hospital that I don't like."

"What deal?" Dolores perked up. She was on the medical executive committee, a collection of doctors that interfaced between the hospital management functions and the professional responsibilities of the doctors on the medical staff. Part of that was monitoring agreements that affected the two entities.

"They get upset when I expose their plans. Plus, they don't tell me anything since I gave notice."

"You're kidding."

"They tried to fire me for cause last week for saying something to a corporate attorney." "Wow."

"I have a ton of money in the practice. They keep it if I get fired for cause. Ergo, I must,

behave myself."

"The golden handcuffs."

"Something like that."

She ignored what she thought was Harrison's hyperbole. He was known for bold statements. "Are you going to start Thompson on steroids?"

"No. The Myocarditis Trial established there was no clinical benefit."

"Biopsy?"

"No benefit, according to that trial."

"So, do we just wait?"

"I started a beta blocker. There are no data that it works or doesn't but it helps with heart failure in general. She might not be able to tolerate it even in tiny amounts. We'll see."

"The abdominal pain is from liver distention due to heart failure, is that what you think?"

"That or referred pain from her heart."

"Hugh, I'm not sure I have much to add here. It seems to be all cardiac."

"I agree."

"Great. I'll let you run the show but I'll see her every day." She moved away to chart.

Harrison looked at the bank of monitors, tired and sleep deprived. His eyes closed, the present faded and a memory emerged.

"We met with the administrator of Saint Lucius Medical Center before Christmas," said Sarisha Malouf, leading a meeting months earlier. "They have offered us six thousand square feet or more of office space attached to the hospital. They need us there, so I think we could get a better rental rate if we wanted it. I told them we might be interested."

There was a murmur of discontent. Monty Pierce spoke up. "I'm not at all interested, personally. We have a large office here at OCHA and our own cath lab. It makes no sense to pay more rent."

Malouf never tilted away from the table and folded her arms, waiting for more discussion. The tiny space between her front teeth sometimes made her smile ominous. Lebanese olive skin, black hair and her oval face reminded Hugh of a cat.

"When it opens, will Saint Luce have access to insurance plans that OCHA does not?" Stan Blackstone asked from beneath his bushy brows.

"That's what they say," Malouf purred, "but that's up in the air."

"When we talked about this a while ago, I thought we all wanted some competition for OCHA," Harrison said, then noticed Jennifer Hayes standing tall and close to the glass doors, waiting to be invited in. She watched the proceedings unable to hear the dialogue.

"We did," Malouf said. "But it's major threat to OCHA, our primary hospital. You're on the Board of Saint Lucius, Hugh, and that puts us in an awkward position here."

"We think you should resign from the Board, Hugh," said Pierce. His bushy gray walrus mustache, full head of salt-and-pepper hair, deep lines in a tanned heavy face and his smooth voice lured many into believing he knew what he was talking about.

"We?" Hugh asked with a challenge. "Two years ago, you wanted me to get involved with the company."

"That was then and before I sat in this chair," said Malouf. "Your involvement gets in the way of a close relationship with OCHA."

"It was in our best interest to have board members on the hospitals where we practice," Hugh argued. "Monty is on the board of Sam's. Nigel is at on the board here."

"Jennifer Hayes and I have discussed options that would change our relationship with Olympus." The pitch of Malouf's voice dropped half a step.

"Like what?"

"We can't tell you anything if you are on their Board, Hugh," Pierce rumbled.

"I'm a shareholder here. You can't keep stuff like that away from me."

"You have a conflict of interest," Blackstone decreed.

Hugh looked at the faces in the room. Half a dozen were averted. The rest looked down on him with disdain.

"I think it's a great thing to be starting a hospital that is geared toward superior service, great medical care and relationships with docs where incentives are aligned, where the financial goal is not giving the investors more return but plowing profit back into the facility for continuous improvements. I like the concept. I'd rather not resign."

"We cannot discuss the OCHA opportunities with you present," Malouf said as she glanced toward Hayes, waiting for the invitation to enter. "It's up to you."

"Why the secrecy?"

"It's propriety information they want to keep away from competitors," Sarisha explained.

"I'll resign," Harrison said after a short pause. "Not from Saint Luc', from here." He stood, collected a small sheaf of papers from the table and moved to the door in a glass wall. "While I don't know exactly what you've been up to, it doesn't smell good. I'm tired of your petty politics. This is no longer the practice I want to be in. You'll have my letter of resignation in the morning." He left the room, nodding to Jennifer, who passed him on her way inside.

"We'll be looking forward to it," Malouf said as he left.

The rhythm lines came back into focus as the memory faded. His ongoing nightmare was swept underneath the crush of patients needing him. He went to see Thompson.

CHAPTER 7

"Mommy!" Amy ran in and belly-flopped onto the bed.

Sarah pulled her up by the armpits and hugged. A thin, bald, smiling grandfather and a plump scowling grandmother soon followed.

"She is a handful," Myra Szabo said.

"Hi, Mom, Dad."

"You look darn good for being sick," Myra said, looking good herself with dark brown, lustrous curled hair inconsistent with the age of her face. Lipstick too red, mascara too thick and make-up too blush.

"I don't feel too bad as long as I lie here in bed," she countered.

"I've felt that same way all my life," Ed Szabo joked.

No one laughed. His rim of gray hair made him look older than sixty-five. His yellowed toothed smile disappeared quickly as the women talked.

"Happy, happy," cooed Amy, burying her face into Sarah's chest.

"Thanks for bringing Amy. Did you have trouble with Doug?"

"Not a bit," Myra said. "He probably was happy to have the night off. I told him she would stay with us tonight."

"Are you sure?"

"She's a little firecracker but we'll do just fine. What did your doctor say today?"

"They were both by this morning. I had another heart test but I don't know what it showed."

"Well, that's not right."

"It's a weekend, Mom. Things probably run a bit slower."

"This is a hospital, not a dry cleaner. You should have service around the clock. Ed, go ask the nurse for the test results."

She shooed him away with a fluttering hand and fingers. He hesitated and caved in without argument since he never won if he tried. He slipped out the door.

"I'd like to talk to your doctor," Myra continued with little pause. "I want to know what's going on. I hate secrets."

"It's seven o'clock on a Saturday night. They have personal lives. Leave them alone."

"Aren't they on duty? If they're working then they should be available to tell you about your test. Lord knows they are paid enough. They are probably having a spa treatment, sipping iced Perrier with lime surrounded by New Age music and half-naked women."

"Mom, you are a riot." Sarah laughed.

"I'm serious."

"That's what's so funny."

"Don't laugh at me."

"I can't help it. You live in some world that doesn't exist and it amazes me. I work with a lot of doctors. That's not how most of them live."

"I hope they pay you well."

"I can afford to give you and Dad a thousand dollars a month."

That hit a nerve. Myra withdrew, pursed her lips and folded her arms. "We're not your charity cases, my dear."

"Not at all. But, Dad's income is not much. As long as I can afford it, it's fine for me to support you. After all, you supported me for twenty years."

"We certainly did."

Ed returned.

"Well?" Myra stared at him, grateful to have a different topic.

"It's shift change and the nurses are busy."

"The nerve!" Myra moved to the opposite side of the room and wiggled into a stuffed chair.

"What did you do today?" Sarah asked Amy, who had sat up and started to inspect the TV control box. She petted Amy's face and hair.

Almost an hour later, the redheaded Aaron entered, on duty again. The talk had dried up.

Ed leaned against the wall, tired of standing and of living in his personal existential hell. "It's me again," he said with a wry grin. "Back for another night shift. Do you need anything?"

"Young man," Myra began.

"Stop, Mom." Her mother obeyed but fumed. "Do you have the result of the scan from this morning?"

"Yes," he said as he unfolded a piece of paper. "I heard it in report. Let's see. Ejection fraction was 42 percent."

"Thanks, Aaron," Sarah said.

"If there's nothing else, I'll be back soon." He left in a hurry.

"What is 42 percent?" Myra asked. "That doesn't sound so good."

Amy pulled tissues out of a box slowly and laid them in an emesis basin one on top of another, turning each one so that the corners made a star pattern.

"It's a measure of the strength of my heart."

"You only have forty-two percent of your heart working?"

"That's not what it means. They said normal is fifty percent."

"I wish I could talk to your doctor."

"They come by in the mornings. They tell me everything. I don't know that they would tell you anything different."

"Doctors keep the bad news away from patients."

"Maybe they used to. Dr. Barton has always been very open and honest. She's great."

"I just don't know what to think about women doctors and male nurses. It seems upside down." Myra fussed and adjusted her position in the chair. "What about the heart specialist?"

"I don't know him as well but he seems good."

"He better be," Ed said under his breath.

"What was that, Ed?"

"Nothing. Just mumbling." Aaron put a folding chair in the room and left again without a word.

Someone cares, Ed thought as he sat.

"I need a restroom," Myra said, rocking and shifting until she could extract her ample hips from the arms that clung to her generous rump. She walked out.

"I'm worried about you," Ed said.

"Me, too," she said. "It's scary."

"Reminds me of when you were riding down Millcreek Canyon in the dark, hit someone and went flying from your bike. You broke your skull. I was certain you'd never be the same."

"Maybe I got dumb enough to become a CPA instead of an attorney."

Ed laughed. "The only dumb thing you did was marry the loser."

"I'll blame that on the bike accident."

"It was an accident of some sort."

"You didn't marry very well, yourself, Dad."

His eyes moistened.

"But you stuck with it. Better than I could do."

"Part of that is a generation thing. And Doug is an unmitigated disaster. Never should have married him."

"I was pregnant."

"So?"

Amy left her mother's bed and hugged Ed, her head against his chest. She said nothing.

"We're sculpted by our mistakes," Ed said.

"And Mom has chipped away so much stone from you that there's hardly anything left, Dad. Why do you stay with her?"

He looked out the door, then back at Amy then back to Sarah. "I made a promise, honey."

"You deserve happiness," Sarah said. "I love you both but how you two ever got together and stayed together is one of the mysteries of the world."

A few minutes later the three visitors left, leaving Sarah alone for another night in the hospital. Her dad's last statement still in her head. "Tell you what. When you get completely better, I'll retire and help take care of the little urchin."

CHAPTER 8

A cloth gown with ties, not snaps, was bunched up covering only Sarah's chest. Blankets were pulled down to her knees. A thin blue towel was folded about three inches wide and covered her privates. She looked nervous and cold. Laci, an outgoing technologist, chatted at her, making widening circles over the junction of her thigh and abdomen with a sponge stick loaded with germicide. Debbie, a nurse, emptied two syringes of sedation into the IV that fed into the left arm, telling Laci with her crusty gaze to shut up. Laci went on about life in Logan, Hyrum and Paradise, towns located ninety miles north. Harrison scrubbed his hands and watched. In a minute, Sarah was asleep.

"I used to biopsy all these patients," Hugh said toward the end of the procedure, looking at the black and white screen, holding a plastic three-ring syringe and three port manifold. "I would have biopsied her today but that's no longer the recommendation. Some would call it malpractice if I did since there's a small risk with it. There are probably some that are certain that failing to biopsy is malpractice."

Laci manipulated a joystick and the X-ray tube assembly moved. "I think the last biopsies we did were with you a couple of years ago."

"That sounds about right."

"So, Hugh, do you think she has myocarditis?" Laci was comfortable using first names of physicians. Her shoulder length brown hair was tucked unto a disposable blue bouffant hat. A surgical mask and protective X-ray glasses hid her thin face and pleasantly crooked nose. Her large brown eyes and long lashes peaked over the surgical mask hopefully with the same seductive effect of wearing a veil.

"I do." He injected contrast and took another cine. "Clean arteries, as expected in a young woman."

Laci moved the X-ray tube as he refilled his syringe.

She wanted to sleep with Harrison, just once, to see what he was like. It was out of curiosity, for no other reason. His personality was fun; his face was not. She imagined a flabby chest and belly. He was single and should have been an easy target. Not so easy after all.

They took the final picture. He deftly inserted a tuft of collagen into the needle tract to stop bleeding, launched his rubber gloves into a red trash bin. In the control room he traced the pictures of the left ventricle. The ejection fraction was 38 percent. Warm paper fed out of the laser printer. Harrison reviewed the pressures and flows. Her heart was pumping less blood flow than normal but it was not a severe decrease. Sarah had been moved to a stretcher and was talking groggily when he approached.

"No blocked arteries, as we thought," he told her, his hand on her shoulder to make her more awake.

"Is that good?"

"Yes and no. Your heart muscle is weak, probably inflamed. Most people get better quickly but you haven't turned around quite yet."

Laci stood too close to Hugh, pressing against the back of his right arm until the conversation ended. She and Debbie wheeled Sarah out of the lab and back to her room.

Harrison was dictating the catheterization report in a darkened film review room when Sedi, another experienced nurse, came in. She spoke with urgency. "Could you come next door?"

"Hold on," he said then finished his paragraph. He put the phone down. "What's up?"

"Tombstone perforated a coronary," she spoke slowly to compensate for her Persian accent. "The patient's crashing. We need you in there now." The staff's nickname for Blackstone made him cringe even though at times like this it seemed well earned.

"Did he ask you to get me?"

"No, but you know he never asks for help, he just lets his patients die."

Hugh exhaled in frustration and followed Sedi next door. It looked like a fire drill. Chaos. Shouting. Too many people, too little leadership. A middle aged guy with shaved head and Brillo pad facial hair was "bagging" the patient, making her breathe as he clamped a face mask over her nose and mouth. He was getting excessively radiated as Blackstone focused on his work. Blood pressure almost nil. Heart rate twice normal. Two nurses hanging IV bags with red lettering and dialing in doses on computerized pumps. Scrub table cluttered. Wrappers strewn on the floor, garbage can trash overflowing, taking over the area, threatening to fill the room. Panic sucking oxygen away from everyone, seen under the bushy brows of Blackstone.

"You need any help, Stan?" Harrison asked twice before getting a response. "Everything's fine here," he said.

The two nurses threw disgusted stares of disbelief.

"I beg to differ," said the more experienced, older nurse, Megan. "Her pressure is in the crapper. She needs to be intubated and needs a pericardiocentesis."

"She'll be fine as soon as I get this covered stent deployed," he said. "We are almost there."

"Her pressure is 50/30," Megan countered. "After three milligrams of Epi' and on Levophed."

"You'll never get the stent past this bend," said Pete, who was scrubbed and assisting. "It's almost there," Blackstone growled. "We're fine and I don't need help!"

Hugh moved into the control booth where he could watch everything. The blip-blip of the ECG turned into a random scribble and the blood pressure line settled into flat at thirty-five. "V fib!" the monitor tech next to Hugh shouted into the microphone.

Blackstone and Pete looked up. Megan was already at the defibrillator.

Within seconds she punched the charge button and a whistle raised in pitch and volume. Large patches had been stuck on the lady earlier.

"Clear!" Megan said.

Blackstone kept working, foot on the fluoroscopy pedal. Everyone else had back off, hand in the air.

"Clear!" she said again. "Dr. Blackstone, that means you."

He kept working. She hit the lighted button and the lady arched in a titanic twitch.

"What the—?" Blackstone shouted. "You could have shocked me. I was not clear."

The rhythm returned to its previous pattern and the blood pressure returned near 50.

Sedi came into the control booth. "Isn't there something you can do?"

"You heard him, he does not want me in there."

"This shit is why we call him Tombstone," the monitor tech softly interjected.

"Call Ted Hatcher. He's the medical director," Harrison said. "And call anesthesia. If someone shows up, Blackstone will allow the patient to be intubated at least."

Sedi started calling when the patient's rhythm returned to fibrillation. The tech called it out again and Harrison went back into the room. The defibrillator whined again.

Megan called out, "CLEAR! Damn it!"

Blackstone looked at her angrily. "Watch your language!"

She punched the button and dispensed fifty thousand volts.

"I'm going to report you," he said. "Wait until I'm clear before you shock."

"Stop ignoring me!"

"Amiodarone one hundred fifty milligrams bolus," Harrison said.

Blackstone glowered. "Try putting in a buddy wire," he offered.

He went to the head of the patient, ranged through a toolkit finding the things he needed. He slipped the curved blade into the unconscious patient's throat, pulled forward and placed a breathing tube into the trachea. The bearded therapist listened to both lungs and Harrison looked at the fluoroscopic image to confirm the tube was feeding the correct organs. The therapist pumped oxygen in large volumes into the starving lungs. Numbers improved.

On the screen, the additional wire jerked and twitched clumsily down the coronary. The covered stent then went past the bend. However, no contrast could pass and the location of the perforation was no longer apparent.

"You should do a pericardiocentesis, Stan," Hugh advised. "Pressure is still fifty. She'll be brain dead soon if she's not already."

"I thought I asked you to leave."

"Somebody's gotta take care of the patient," he said.

"Get out."

"Relieve the tamponade. Otherwise, this is an assassination."

"What's up?" Ted Hatcher walked in wearing street clothes, no hat, no mask.

"Coronary perforation," Blackstone said. "I have a covered stent ready to deploy and Harrison is interfering with the procedure and endangering my patient. He refuses to leave."

"Why don't you step outside, Hugh." It was not a question.

Hatcher stayed in the room. Sedi handed him a kit for pericardiocentesis. Three heads in the room shook in disbelief as Harrison exited. The monitor tech put both hands up and open, eyebrows raised. Hopeless. Sedi followed him out.

"Thank you for coming," she said.

His next patient had been wheeled into the room. No time for anger. "It's so good to feel wanted," he replied.

CHAPTER 9

A wooden tray with freshly sliced sourdough bread, Italian salami, pear, apple and cheeses sat on Harrison's rustic dining table. A single lamp hanging low provided the only source of light, awash over the food and spilling into the kitchen. Ashleigh Ashe, in jeans and a red-brown Kokopelli T-shirt had fixed a simple meal. She uncorked a Fisher-Cameron blend as Hugh lumbered in from the garage. Her long, slender bare feet were silent on the wood floor. Her oblong face ended in a tapering chin and was framed with medium brown hair curling off her shoulders. Blue-green eyes met Hugh's adoring gaze from the entry.

"How are things at Holladay High?" he asked.

"Just another parade of high school English classes," she sighed. "No fights, no drugs today."

"Where are Bret and Ben?"

"With Cal." Her two boys, eleven and thirteen, were staying with her ex-husband, an electrical contractor with a growing business. "You've got to be tired after three nights of call."

"Yep. Tuckered out," he mimicked a cheaper western.

He dropped his briefcase in the doorway leading toward the stairs and glided behind Ashleigh, putting his arms around her, smelling her hair, her neck, pulling her tight. She rested her head back, savoring the touch then twisted her neck to find his lips.

"Ummm," she moaned. "It's good to have you home." She had her own house in an older neighborhood but she stayed with Hugh often lately.

"I was here all weekend."

"If you can call it that. On the phone all night, running into the hospital at three in the morning. Or coming home then. I'm not sure how you do it."

"You get used to it."

"Why don't they treat you guys like commercial pilots or long haul truckers? Make you rest and not work sleep deprived."

She sat at the table. He opened the refrigerator and brought out a butter dish.

"There's no FAA for doctors, no rules in private practice. If I lived in some places, I might be the only cardiologist in town, no breaks, always on call."

"When it's late and I'm going over papers, I don't think well," she said. "Don't you make mistakes?"

"Probably more than I know. Most are caught by the nurses. I don't recognize them until I look at a chart when I'm fresh." When first in practice he thought he never erred. How time changes perception, he thought. He scooted his chair closer to Ashleigh. She was beautiful.

"That's scary."

Reggae played softly in the background as a gas log radiated heat and ambience. Fatigue began to settle in his mind like night fog. "How was school?"

"You already asked." She stroked his cheek. "You *are* tired."

"Busy Monday after a weekend of call. Four caths, one defibrillator. No real disasters, at least not of my own. Blackstone was attempting to murder someone that one of the nurses dragged me in to save."

"Did you?"

"I was removed."

"Isn't he dangerous?"

"We reviewed his numbers. He has more complications than any three of us. No one wants to get rid of him, the hospital, the group, the lab director."

"Because he brings in a lot cases."

"Yep." He clinked her wine glass.

They put butter and Brie on French bread, washing it down with wine in a lull of conversation.

"How are your patients doing?" Ashleigh touched his arm.

"I'm a little worried about a young mother. I keep hoping she'll get better but she's not."

"What does she have?"

"Something called myocarditis."

"How old is she?"

"Thirty-four."

"That's not so young."

"She has a nine-year-old girl."

Ashleigh stretched, arched. He was embarrassed when she noticed he was ogling.

"I should trim your eyebrows," Ashleigh said.

He pulled them, measuring and self-conscious. "If they got long enough, I could do a comb-over." His hand gesture simulated a pompadour.

"Good idea. Very attractive." She put the bulbous wineglass to her lips and savored.

He pasted a dollop of Brie on a slice of apple.

"How long have we been dating?" he asked.

"Dating?" She asked putting her glass down, studying his face, as if trying to discern where this was leading. "We saw a play in November, your season tickets, so two and a half years ago."

"Right."

"I don't view our relationship as dating. Do you?"

"No, I'm just not sure what term is appropriate."

"Committed. I was planning on asking you about selling my house and moving the boys and me in. They love your place."

"You should."

She didn't seem to notice his equivocation but he was too sleepy for a meaningful dialogue. He just wanted peace and sleep.

"I'm wasting money on utilities and payments."

"What would your kids think?" The boys were raised in a religion. Formal cohabitation could cause some emotional confusion. Of course, the frequent sleepovers probably already did.

"They brought it up."

"Let's sleep on it." The decision was deferred. He had to resolve his nagging attraction to Jana, the beautiful ultrasound technologist he dated while separated and who left when she got tired of waiting for him to become available. Then he had deal with the aversion acquired in his almost twenty-year marriage to a socialite who had learned to spend money in vast amounts.

CHAPTER 10

During the night the post-cardiac surgical ICU, Blackstone's patient with the perforated artery had no less than eight drugs infusing into her system, a grove of metal poles around the head of the bed supporting the pumps that controlled the infusions.

"Why is it so many of Tombstone's patients end up here, circling the drain?" a thin middle-aged nurse asked about three in the morning.

"The cath lab staff says he has no finesse," replied Dale, the other nurse, as he made adjustments to the console at the foot of the bed.

"Either that or bad judgement. Did you talk to Obi-Poku?"

"That poor guy gets stuck with his disasters. He had me change to a more aggressive insulin regimen and stop the lidocaine drip the surgeon just ordered."

"I can't believe they left this lady's chest open. This is beyond the pale."

"She's alive. She had so much swelling after her surgery that every time they tried to close her—"

"Yeah, I know the story. It's just criminal. How Blackstone does not get sued out of existence is beyond me." She flicked her straight brown hair out of her face.

"God is on his side. "

"Dale, don't get me started on that."

In the morning the patient had survived a withering barrage of cardiac arrests and prolonged periods without adequate blood pressure. Outside the bay where his patient lay, Blackstone, in scrubs, spoke with a neurologist wearing a suit. He explained he could not assess her brain condition until the medications were tapered. As Harrison passed nearby, Blackstone ignored him. The neurologist recommended continuing the cooling blankets and the induced coma for at least one more day. One of the two nurses from the night shift mouthed the word "help" as Harrison passed on his way out. He shrugged a "what can I do?" and gestured with his thumb toward Blackstone.

Harrison had six patients to see on CTU in the two hours before a scheduled pacemaker. Sarah's chart showed unchanged labs and vital signs. Her rhythm had been normal, an improvement. He entered her room to find her alone and dozing.

"Hey there," he said as he rubbed her foot through a homemade quilt with an unusual more contemporary design and bright yellows and reds. Her lids flipped open.

"Good morning." She yawned and twisted. "I didn't sleep well."

"No one does around here. The hospital's no place to be if you're sick." She managed a wee smile. "How does your chest feel?"

"It's fine. It's never bothered me. It's confusing that my heart's messed up but feels fine but my stomach hurt. It hasn't bothered me for a day or two."

He listened to her lungs and heart, poked at her liver and shins, studied her neck. Her jugular veins were still plump with the excess burden of heart failure. As he examined her, he noticed several photographs of family on the counter. One looked like a parody of the classic *American Gothic* painting by

Grant Wood, absent the pitchfork and that the woman was adorned with overdone makeup.

"Things look about the same today. No improvement but no worsening either. I think we'll just keep on with the same medication. I'd like to increase the dose but your blood pressure is still pretty low."

"So, I'm not going home today, then?"

"No, I'm sorry."

"I just sit around in the hospital taking pills twice a day?"

"It's not safe to send you home. You still get lightheaded when you get out of bed, right?"

"Sometimes, yeah."

"And you have no one at home that could help take care of you?"

"It's just my daughter and I. She's nine."

"Is that your girl?" He pointed at one of the photos.

"That's my little Amy."

"Who are these people?" He put a finger on the Gothic photo.

Sarah laughed. "Don't you just love that picture. They are my parents. I wanted to have some fun so I had them dress up for the picture. My dad's face is so, gosh, unexpressive. He looks like he never had a day of fun in his whole life but behind the mask is or was a fun guy. My mom had to smear on theatrical lipstick, rouge and color her hair like she was a stage actress. I think it captured my parents' personalities so well and they have no idea. None." She laughed again followed by a series of coughs.

"We'll see how you do today. We'll do another heart test tomorrow. I'd like to see your heart function stabilize or improve."

"Another angiogram?"

"No. A MUGA. The radioactive test that we did a couple of days ago."

"That wasn't bad."

"You just have to lie there with your arms over your head. Pretty easy."

"Did you know the nurses here respect you?"

"They would never tell me that."

"They say I have the best cardiologist in town."

"That's very flattering. What you really have is the nicest quilt in the hospital. Did you make it?"

"Yes. It's a relaxing pastime." She cleared her throat. "They say you are not only a good doctor but a good person. It gives me faith that you're doing your best."

Hugh looked down.

She reached forward and took his right hand. "Thank you. Thank you very much." "You're welcome," he responded uncomfortably. He left a moment later.

A little after three in the afternoon, in the middle of his office clinic schedule, Harrison's pager chirped. It was the number to the CTU. He called.

"Sarah passed out," a nurse named Lindsay said with a little alarm in her voice. "She had tried to walk five short steps to the bathroom and ended up on the floor, stooping over first before she lost consciousness because she felt it coming on. Her heart monitor showed a little increase in rate but nothing else. Her blood pressure was seventy-two before we got her back to bed." Lindsay took a deep breath after the rapid report.

"That's not good," he replied.

"Do you want to order anything?"

"You have a hold order on her carvedilol for hypotension, right?"

"Not to give if her pressure is less than 85."

"Good enough," he said.

The call ended but his concern intensified.

Jennifer Hayes stood when Dr. Malouf whisked in to her office wearing a white coat over black slacks and an orange silk blouse. Hayes' hand dwarfed Sarisha's as they shook to start the conversation.

"This is cardiac cath lab contract," Jennifer said as she handed her a folder.

"I'll have Jon Gullimore, our attorney, look at it. Are there any surprises or changes since we last spoke?" She pulled out a sheaf of papers and began to flip through it.

"We made it a three-year agreement. The pay is covered in Appendix B." Jennifer turned there in Sarisha's copy, putting a finger on each line.

"We wanted five years."

"It automatically renews."

They chatted for several minutes about details.

"You understand this is confidential," Hayes said.

"I know that."

"Specifically, we don't want Saint Lucius to have even an inkling we are negotiating."

"Right."

"You will keep this away from Harrison, then?"

"He probably knows we are negotiating with you about something, that's it."

Blackstone walked in. "Sorry I'm late," he mumbled.

"Take a seat," Malouf said.

"We can't afford Harrison messing this thing up," Hayes continued after handing Blackstone a copy. "If he does, it could kill the deal."

"He's leaving soon, plus I have Gullimore working on ways to fire him for cause and get him out even sooner. We'll keep him out of the loop. He'll be out of town for our next meeting when we'll discuss this in detail with our attorney's comments and the financial projections."

"Good," she responded, then hesitated. "There's a part of our agreement that will not find its way onto paper. You understand that, right?"

"Absolutely," Sarisha said.

"What's that?" Blackstone asked.

"That none of us will practice at Saint Lucius," Sarisha said.

"That's not in here?" Blackstone looked through the numbered and lettered paragraphs.

"Only in the sense that we can terminate the agreement with one hundred twenty days' notice without cause," Hayes pointed out.

"Has your corporate legal department in Houston looked at this?" Sarisha asked.

"They'll see the final version. Local counsel drafted this."

"It does not expose us to any legal problems?"

"We would not propose it if we thought there was any question but talk to your own attorney. You don't have to enter into the agreement. We lose a lot of money to do this and your group benefits richly from our effort to kill Auspicious Health. If you don't sign it won't affect our relationship with your group moving forward. Remember, you came to us with this, not the other way around."

"Got it," Sarisha said.

"I might be able to sideline Harrison," said Blackstone out of nowhere. "I can get him in some difficulty with the medical staff because his behavior."

Don Zone frequently referred to Blackstone as a useful idiot. Hayes thought he was half right. She did not express her skepticism. "As long as he doesn't get in the way of this agreement, I'm happy. Is there anything you want to discuss now or shall we wait until you've had a chance to go over the language?"

"You and I should talk sometime before our group meeting," Malouf offered as she stood, the signal that the meeting had concluded.

Blackstone stayed in his seat, reading the agreement. Hayes, towering over Malouf, shook her limp little hand with a firm squeeze before she left. Blackstone startled, saw that his partner had departed and hurried out.

CHAPTER 11

Harrison heard Dr. Dolores Barton's coarse, deep voice when he walked in to the CTU. She was arguing on the phone. She slid Thompson's chart in his direction.

The computer yielded lab values and a graph of Sarah's vital signs. Over the last four days she had been given about half of the doses of carvedilol, the beta-blocking drug he had ordered. Nurses had withheld it for low blood pressure. Her heart rate was perhaps better, seventy-five, and most of her systolic blood pressures were between ninety and one hundred. They were always measured with her lying in bed.

Dolores crashed the phone down, took off her stylish, skinny glasses and rubbed her eyes. "Partner troubles," she said. "But you wouldn't know anything about that, would you, Hugh?" She didn't smile.

"Never have a moment's trouble with my group." He laughed.

Now she smiled just a bit. "You compete with your college friends to get into med school. You gun in school for residencies, trying to one-up everyone. When you're there, you joust for the best recommendations. You'd think we'd all tire of the stupid games. It never freaking ends. Now it's about time or money."

"Usually both."

"Anyway, I just saw Thompson. She seems to be going nowhere. What's your plan?"

"Her ejection fraction fell again. I wasn't expecting that."

"But that's why you look."

"Right. I might refer her to the heart failure clinic uptown."

"Why wait?"

"They like to enroll patients in studies. That's fine except most of their research treatments increase mortality rates. I'm hoping the beta blocker will work but it hasn't had enough time."

"Funny how it was hammered into us for years they should not be used in heart failure," Barton said.

"Europeans were using beta blockers for decades and they worked. Most Americans just started five or six years ago."

"When will you get another ejection fraction?"

"Saturday, unless I transfer her."

"I'll be off."

"I'll be out of town, too." He returned the chart to her. "I'm going to let her know what we found."

Harrison contemplated how to deliver the news as he approached the door. Sarah was alone.

"I don't think I've ever met your family." He nodded at the *American Gothic* picture. "Do they come to visit?"

She turned from the television screen and fumbled for the volume control. "I'm sorry, what did you say?"

He repeated the question.

"My daughter is coming with my parents. They visit every night."

"If I'm here late, I'll try to come in and meet them. I looked at the scan. Your heart has not improved. Your ejection fraction is slightly lower, thirty-five percent. That's still not too bad but it keeps falling. Five days ago it was forty-two percent using the same test."

"Are you going to keep me here?"

"I'm sorry."

"The hospital is nice and the people are friendly. The service is great. I just want to be home, that's all."

"I'm thinking of referring you to a heart failure program. If your heart gets weaker you may need some of their specialized work."

"Really? This is a good heart program here."

"It's great but we don't offer advanced therapies here."

"What kind of advanced therapies?"

"They have research medications and surgical treatments such as heart transplant or ventricular assist devices."

"Transplant? Am I going to need that?"

"I don't know that you will need one but if your number keeps falling, it will be on the list of treatments. This disease, as I think I told you, usually gets better on its own without treatment. A few people have progressive heart failure and need a new heart."

"I could die from this?"

"Some people do."

"My daughter needs me. My ex is a disaster and my parents are too old to raise another kid, especially one with special needs." She reached for the tissue box, pulled out a couple, dabbed her eyes dry.

"What's wrong with your girl?" Harrison asked, although he thought he knew the answer.

"Down syndrome. She does pretty well. She's able to go to school but I don't know if she'll ever be totally independent."

Barton entered.

Sarah looked at her as she dabbed at both eyes. "He said I could die from this," Sarah sniffled.

"Yes, but that's rare these days," Barton said as she sat on edge of the bed.

Sarah reached up; Dolores bent down and hugged her. Sarah sobbed. Harrison backed off, feeling like he had been cruel. He remembered a Mark Twain short story about the virtue of lying how it's sometimes impossible to be both honest and kind.

"I can't leave my daughter alone. I can't. I can't," she repeated over and again.

"You'll get better," Barton said. "Whatever it takes. You'll get through this and see your little Amy grow old, older than you are now."

"I'm officially scared," Sarah said, wiping her eyes.

"It's hard when you have to face your own mortality, especially when you have so much to live for," Barton said.

"I love her so much," she sobbed.

"I can tell."

She laughed through her tears then straightened up. "I never cry in front of strangers. I'm so embarrassed."

"There are no strangers here, Sarah." Barton stood. "No one is more concerned about you than we. Both of us. Well, at least I am."

That brought another soft smile. Sarah, the patient, the mom, the accountant and all the other representations of her essence, looked with watery, red eyes at her two physicians, the caring internist at the foot of the bed and cardiologist with a bad mustache standing a foot behind. "Amy needs me. God would not, will not let her grow up with her sleazy father or alone in the world. I will make it through this."

"We expect you to get better, Sarah," Harrison said.

"If I don't, I'll come back to haunt you."

"All the more reason to get you well," Barton said. "He has plenty of women pestering him."

All three of them laughed.

A few minutes later the two doctors conversed at the nursing station.

"I have a daughter about the same age as Sarah's girl," Dolores said. "I can hardly imagine how terrified she must be. I have a husband who is a good dad. Amy's father is a loser, a horrible personality disorder."

"I hope Sarah turns the corner in the next couple of days. I'll be gone for the first half of next week. I'd like to see her improving before I leave."

"See you later, Hugh," she said as she left.

He made a note reminding him to call Bill Ward, a heart failure specialist uptown tomorrow.

CHAPTER 12

The next day, Thursday, Harrison's pager buzzed with the number to the CTU as he walked from his car to the office. He called back from his desk. "Harrison."

"This is Raven. Thompson in fifteen passed out again this morning after getting out of bed."

"What was her rhythm?"

"Sinus. Rate was 130. Her pressure was ninety-one over fifty-four by the time we got her back in bed."

"Was she injured?"

"She hit her head. Probably not bad but we should get a CT scan."

"Is she confused?"

"She's sharper than me. But I've been up all night."

"Sharper than I."

"I doubt it."

Harrison smiled. "I'll check her in a few minutes."

"She might be in CT."

"I haven't ordered it."

"It's protocol. We have to get a head CT on falls when a patient hits their head."

Harrison ended the call then called Wasatch Heart Failure Clinic and got his old friend on the phone, a cardiologist specializing in heart failure and transplants.

"Dr. Ward," he announced.

"Hey, Bill, this is Hugh Harrison."

"A blast from the past. What's up?" His response was cool.

"I need to run a case by you. A thirty-four-year-old woman was admitted with belly pain but had elevated MB. A week ago her heart function was mildly reduced, ejection fraction forty-eight percent as I recall. On beta blocker her ejection fraction has fallen to thirty-five percent. Normal coronaries, so probably acute myocarditis. Stable heart rate in the nineties at rest, systolics in the eighties and nineties. Is this someone I should transfer to you?"

"What are her symptoms now?"

"She has passed out several times. Probably orthostatic hypotension since her heart rate is high when that happens."

"Stop the beta blocker first," he said after asking a few more questions. "Give her a few days and if she's the same or worse, we should move her here."

"It'll be the weekend."

"We're open. I'll be off but someone will be working. She might need a biopsy."

"I thought that was no longer part of the workup."

"It's not, at least not usually. But in her we might need to rule out a couple of kinds of myocarditis that require special treatments. Based on what you said, we can probably wait."

"Aren't you about ready to retire?" Harrison asked.

"I'm old enough that I don't take night call anymore. I'll probably hang it up next year."

Harrison ordered another heart scan for Friday hoping he could see it before he left town.

Friday marked one week of Sarah's hospitalization. She celebrated by pushing a wheelchair once around the nursing station, slowly and without fainting. The chair was good support plus a quick way back to home base if she felt puny. A nuclear technologist drew her blood when she stopped. By midmorning the test was done.

"Your ejection fraction was down to thirty-three percent," Harrison explained around midday. She was still pale but otherwise looking good. "It's hard to say if that is a real decrease or within the margin of error for the test."

"I walked around the nurse's station this morning," was her response. "It felt good."

"I hope your heart is on the mend."

"So do I. Positive thoughts. Lots of prayer."

"I will be gone for the weekend. I won't be back until Thursday. Dr. Blackstone will be on duty and covering my patients."

"Oh. Okay. I think Dr. Barton has the weekend off, too. I'm sure you both deserve a vacation."

"Unfortunately, I have to go to a meeting, so it's a break but not a vacation."

Her physical exam was the same. Her lab values were stable. She had a minor alteration in heart rhythm early Thursday morning but nothing worrisome. Harrison had not stopped the beta blocker and she had received the last three doses since her blood pressure was reasonable and Harrison had clarified how he wanted the pills given.

A few minutes later he found Blackstone sitting in his office dictating chart notes. He waited, not wanting to interrupt. For a moment he looked forward to the time when he wouldn't have to entrust his patients to him and regretted that he had failed to move him out of the practice.

"I have a flight at about four today," Harrison said when he finished. "I'll be leaving early. Looks like you're on for the weekend. Here's my list." Seven names were handwritten with room numbers and a sketch of the clinical situation. "Sarah Thompson is a thirty-four-year-old CPA with an acute myocarditis," he began to report. "Her ejection fractions have been falling. It was thirty-three percent this morning and thirty-five a couple days earlier. I'm hoping she'll turn around. I ran her by Bill Ward at Wasatch who said he'd accept her in transfer if she didn't improve. I ordered another ejection fraction Monday."

"How are you treating her?"

"Waiting and watching mostly. She is on a tiny dose of carvedilol."

"How do you know it's myocarditis?"

"She had elevated enzymes, normal coronaries and a falling ejection fraction."

"She's been there a week? That's a long time." Harrison shrugged and moved to the next name on the list.

Ashleigh hurried from her last class so she could drop Harrison off at the airport.

"I put my house on the market today," she said with excitement as she drove on I-80 to the airport.

"I thought we were going to talk about this a little more."

"I thought you were okay with us moving in?"

"That's not what I meant."

"We're talking now," Ashleigh said. "What do you think?"

He could deal with physicians, nurses, patients and all kinds of people outside his tight personal life. He froze when he hit intimate conversations.

"Talk to me, Hugh. Say something."

"I worry about how your boys will react to this situation."

"They're happy that I'm happy. And your huge TV is a hit."

"When will you move in?"

"This weekend, while you're gone. I'm going to leave furniture in the house. It'll sell better." She exited the freeway onto the airport road.

"Have you looked into renting it furnished?"

"You don't seem too enthused about this. Do you not want us to move in?"

"I was only thinking you might like some monthly income from the rent."

"Not a bad idea, actually. I'll look into it."

She dropped him off. Inside the terminal he found Debbie, his research nurse, noticeable for her large blonde hair, bright red lipstick and silky, retro clothes. He never looked forward to trips with her as all she could talk about were lab rats that she saved and all the problems of finding sitters, gear and people to adopt them.

CHAPTER 13

Eight-thirty Saturday morning, after looking over Thompson's chart, Stan Blackstone had a mission. She had languished in the hospital for over a week and it was past time to take action. A nurse approached him and asked, "Is 15 being transferred to Wasatch today, Stan?"

The irritation of calling him by his given name rose in his throat. "Not to Wasatch, to the ICU. She needs different meds."

"Dr. Harrison said he talked to a transplant doc at Wasatch."

"I can fix her. She'll do better on the correct treatment." He stood up and walked to room fifteen as she rolled her eyes.

There was a girl lying on the bed with the patient, a heavy woman ensconced in the easy chair and an old guy leaning up against the wall.

"Hello. I'm Dr. Blackstone, the cardiologist," he said with a smile.

"We finally get to meet the doctor," said Myra, not moving. "I have questions." She looked him over suspiciously.

"I'm Sarah and this is my daughter, Amy."

Amy cuddled closer to her mom.

"I'm her mother. Sarah has been here for over a week," Myra continued. "I don't know what's wrong with her, I've never met the doctors and I don't see any progress."

"Dr. Harrison never spoke with you?"

"No," Myra was indignant. "We have been completely ignored."

"Mom," Sarah countered. "You don't visit until evening, after he has gone."

"Her heart is weak," Blackstone explained, focusing on Myra and using hand gestures. "And getting weaker. The negligible treatment she has been getting has done nothing." He glanced infrequently at Sarah but directed his remarks to Myra. "I think we need to take the bull by the horns and jumpstart her heart function."

Sarah knit her brows. Blackstone sensed some doubt or resistance.

"That sounds better than just waiting for something to happen," Myra replied. "Why haven't you done this before now?"

"This is the first time I've seen your daughter. Dr. Harrison has been in charge until today."

"He has the weekend off, Mom," interjected Sarah. "Dr. Blackstone, did you talk this over with him?"

"I would like to transfer you to the intensive care unit, place a couple of lines so we can monitor your progress and start you on a heart stimulant called dobutamine. It will make your heart stronger."

"I don't understand why this was not done before," Myra said.

Blackstone seized the opportunity he had waited for. "I don't think that Dr. Harrison had the best interest of your daughter at heart. This is the only way we can make her heart stronger."

"Well, I'll be darned," Myra murmured.

"I'd like to know what Dr. Barton thinks," Sarah said.

"I don't know if she's around," Stan said. "If not, someone is covering for her. I couldn't help but see the Bible on your dresser."

"This last week has been stressful," Sarah said.

"What church do you attend?"

"When I go, it's the First Presbyterian on South Temple."

"I'm going to get this started before it gets too late in the day."

"I'd like to think about it," Sarah said.

"God bless," Blackstone said, then left.

Sarah hit the call button. An aide came quickly. "Could you page Dr. Barton? I need to speak with her."

"I like this doctor," Myra said. "He is a no-nonsense kind of guy. No pussyfooting around. Ed, could you find me some coffee?" She handed him her empty insulated cup.

He was happy to leave. He had noticed a commercial gourmet coffee stand on the first floor.

While he was gone, Dr. Wallace Wren came in. "I was surprised to learn you are still here. I'm covering for Dr. Barton. I heard you had a question."

"The cardiologist covering for Dr. Harrison just came in and wants me to go to the ICU," Sarah said. "I wanted to know what Dr. Barton thought about that."

"She went out of town for the weekend. When we talked last night, she said the cardiologist was in charge of all the heart treatment. I don't think I could tell you more."

"He wants to treat me with something to strengthen my heart."

"In the ICU? There are a couple of IV drugs that stimulate the heart."

"I wonder why Dr. Harrison didn't start it," Sarah asked.

"It is usually used in the sickest of patients. I noticed that your heart function has been falling. Maybe you were not bad enough until now."

"Is Dr. Harrison troubled?" Myra asked.

"He's an excellent doctor. Why?"

"Something that Dr. Blackstone said." Myra shifted uncomfortably.

Wren examined Sarah, who realized that was something Blackstone had neglected to do, and that Harrison did every day. He asked a few more questions, then left.

The coffee appeared, towing Ed silently behind it. The aide soon followed and started bundling up Sarah's things from the closet and bathroom, placing them in plastic bags, endlessly chatting about the beautiful spring weather, how nice it was outside, her friends who were at the sand dunes on four wheelers and motor bikes, drinking and getting sunburned, having a raucous weekend, hoping they would not get hurt because there is no hospital nearby and the closest ones were terrible, staffed by family doctors and no specialists.

Aaron came in after four days off. "We were told to transfer you to the ICU. I hope that's not a surprise."

"It's a relief," said Myra.

"I thought I had to approve," said Sarah.

"Do you?"

"I'm a little apprehensive."

"That's pretty normal," he said as the bed clunked as the wheels started rolling, brake off. Her bags were stuffed on the foot of the bed.

Amy went to get off but Sarah held her on. "We're going for a ride. This will be fun." A smile edged onto her face.

Ed moved out of the way. Myra stayed in the chair until the bed was almost out of the room. Rocking several times she pulled herself up an away, successful on the second attempt.

"You had some time off," Sarah said to the sandy-haired nurse, scratches on his left hand.

"We went climbing for a few days. It's pretty early so we went south for some sandstone towers."

"Climbing like with a rope?"

"Usually. I don't do much free climbing anymore. My girlfriend doesn't like it."

"Does she climb?"

"Oh, yeah. She's really good. She wanted to do ice but we did a lot of that this winter. It's getting a little soft and I was tired of it. So, we did desert."

Into the elevator, her mother lagging. Ed held the door.

"I'm afraid of heights," Sarah offered. She was filled with fear that hit a peak as they left the room where she had spent most of the last week, that had become her cocoon. Now she faced a new and intimidating medical technical arena, procedures, new nurses and a new cardiologist in whom she had not yet developed trust.

"What do you like to do besides tax returns and play with this little cutie?" Aaron rubbed the top of Amy's head.

"I'm not little."

"We quilt, don't we, Mom?"

"We certainly do," Myra confirmed.

"I glaze and fire small clay figurines and Christmas ornaments. I have my own small kiln."

"It sounds pretty artsy."

"Accounting is very busy between January and April. It's fairly slow in the summer and fall, which is when I do most of the clay. It's a hobby with a little income and good tax breaks." She smiled.

Aaron laughed.

The bed jostled as it rolled over the gap out of the car and onto the second floor. Ceiling and lights passed overhead as she and her daughter looked up, pointing at things. Myra huffed as she struggled to keep up. Ed kept an eye on the stretcher ahead and back at his wife. He collected Amy from the bed at the entrance to the ICU and with the back of one finger stroked Sarah on the cheek, his eyes brimming but trying not to show his own concern. She took his hand and squeezed it. Her bed rolled away. Ed and Amy detoured to the carpeted waiting room in search of a few unoccupied chairs.

A little after noon Blackstone returned to assess the progress of his mission. The catheters were functioning well. Blood pressures inside the various chambers of Sarah's heart were not bad initially. Her amount of blood her heart pumped each minute, called cardiac output, was up to normal now since starting dobutamine. Blackstone was proud. He saw that Myra was pleased with the news.

Sarah's nurse was Jason Jeppson, a guy about her age and a little too similar in appearance to Doug, her ex-husband. However, he was fluid in his movements, confident to the point of almost being bored.

"I feel kind of anxious," she mentioned as he came in for his hourly assessment.

"Sometimes people feel that way on dobutamine."

"Maybe it's just being in the ICU?"

"That could be it."

"It's a dreadful sensation. Dread."

"Really?" Jason looked at the numbers and double checked the drip rates and dosing of the infusion pumps. "Not impending doom, I hope."

"That's kinda what it feels like."

The look on Jason's face darkened. A hollowness grew in her chest. She felt like crying and screaming but remained on her back, looking away from everything and into the ceiling, trying to keep it together.

In the late afternoon a beeping and vibration came from a pager on a belt behind a hedge where Blackstone was measuring, planning to re-landscape the half-acre backyard. He as the extension of the cardiac ICU displayed. He called and spoke with Jason.

"What's up?"

"Mrs. Thompson's breathing rate has gone up to thirty-two and she looks pretty uncomfortable. Her heart rate is one twenty-five. Her wedge pressure is up, twenty-six and her cardiac output has fallen to two-point-five. Would you like me to do anything?"

"Give her forty milligrams of furosemide IV."

"Her pressure is eighty-six."

"Give it anyway."

"Do you want a pulmonologist to see her? Malloy is here."

Stan sighed audibly and intentionally into the phone to give the unspoken message that he didn't need the advice of a nurse. Then he realized if Malloy was involved, he would take over a lot of the care so he wouldn't be bothered. He relented. "I think so, yeah."

"Can I get him on the line for you?"

"Can't you just call him?"

"He's here and he likes doctor-to-doctor communication, like most consultants."

"Alright, get him for me."

The line went to Fogelberg's "Auld Lang Syne" for half a minute.

"Malloy."

"Hi, Les. This is Stan Blackstone. I have a thirty-something-year-old woman with heart failure who might be decompensating. It's probably just a nervous nurse. Her respiratory rate is thirty-two. Could you see her?"

"Sure. No problem. Why does she have heart failure?"

"She has a cardiomyopathy, maybe myocarditis. Her most recent ejection fraction was thirty-three percent."

"Any other medical problems?"

"No."

"I'll go see her in a few minutes."

"Thanks." Stan went back to work with his tape measures and stakes.

A couple hours later Jason entered Sarah's room with a second and larger dose of furosemide, a diuretic that impairs the kidney's ability to hold on to sodium, thus producing prodigious amounts of urine. He was alarmed to see her sitting up, feet dangling off the side, panting. Her face glistened in deathly pallor. A bead of sweat fell from her nose to her knee. She turned toward him, lips blue and eyes wide in fear. The Swan-Ganz catheter appeared to be intact, a major concern when a patient sits up without help. Outside the window was the evil red of sunset.

"Sarah!" he uttered.

He increased the oxygen so high that the prongs up her nose started hissing. She tried to speak but could only manage unintelligible grunts. The monitor showed her oxygen level at 78 percent, heart rate: 145, respiratory rate: 44. He hammered the call button with the edge of his fist. His hand went on her wet back to steady her sway. Her eyes rolled back. She would have collapsed but he steered her back to bed.

Jason called out loudly in the direction of the nursing station. "Need some help in here, now!"

Jennifer O'Toole came in quickly, bringing twenty-five years of ICU experience. After a glance she turned and called from the doorway, "Dr. Malloy, could you come in here?" She hurried to open a plastic bag with an oxygen mask and a second oxygen gauge and popped it into the green receptacle.

Malloy entered and listened to her lungs. "Pulmonary edema. Five milligrams of morphine, IV."

O'Toole hurried out.

Thompson stopped breathing.

The heart monitor showed ten seconds of VT. Malloy grabbed the ventilator bag from Jason. With his left hand he clamped the bad on her nose and mouth and with his right squeezed oxygen into her lungs.

"Stiff," he said. Wet lungs were not easy to inflate.

Alarms beeped. Display flashed. Jason positioned her in the bed. O'Toole returned with a syringe.

"I need to intubate her," Malloy said. She left again to fetch a tackle box that contained all the gear for an emergency intubation. She came back two minutes later.

"Do you have—?" Malloy didn't complete the question because O'Toole held up syringes of a paralyzing drug and a sedative. "Good call. Why am I here?" he asked. "You're the one that gets the big bucks."

"And sued," he said as he assumed control of the intubation kit and Jen administered the paralytic and anesthetic.

A respiratory therapist dashed in and took the bag and mask to control Sarah's breathing. O^2 saturation wallowed in the seventies. Blood pressure flashed dashes, not numbers, unobtainable. Trash accumulated on the floor. Beeping. Another nurse came in. Short statements. Professionals at work. Patient dying.

Within minutes, the crisis eased. Another therapist wheeled in mechanical ventilator. Heart rate and blood pressure improved. O^2 sat was at ninety percent on pure oxygen. Eventually five people in the room dropped to two and then to just Jason. A clump of bags with various meds, ran at precise rates governed by pumps attached to metal poles at the head of her bed. A console controlled her breathing through rubberized accordion white tubing connected to the endotracheal tube that was taped to Sarah's face.

O'Toole found none of Sarah's family in the waiting room, now congested with a Saturday crowd. She paged Dr. Blackstone. Twenty minutes later he called back.

"Mrs. Thompson went into pulmonary edema and had a respiratory arrest," Jason said. "She's on a ventilator." He went over her numbers and drugs. Her cardiac output was low, just under two liters a minute.

"I'll put a balloon pump in her in the morning," he concluded. "I'm glad I started the dobutamine. Looks like I was right to put her in the ICU. It could have been worse."

He made no changes in her medications and gave no other orders. He hung up and raised both arms in triumph. "I am vindicated and Harrison is a moron. His patient crashed, as I predicted and tried to prevent."

His wife, Stacey, seated nearby, folded her book and asked, "Why do you gloat over someone's misfortune?"

"Not gloating. Thankful that God placed that poor soul into my hands, delivered her from the atheist Harrison."

"So, are you going in?"

"We have a pulmonologist there."

"I thought.... Her problem isn't her heart, it's her lungs?" He saw confusion on her face.

"I've got the cardiac situation under control. Her lungs filled up and he can manage that without me there."

She assumed a rather blank look, which he assumed was pride. He had no way of knowing how wrong he was.

Chapter 14

Blackstone dreamed of struggling in a dark green river in turbid turmoil that passed through a huge cement building. Along with his wife and scores of others he splashed and struggled in the irresistible flow. A ringing bell echoed in the halls. Downstream through an ominous hall the river disappeared along with all the people in it into blackness. A second ring.

"Stan!" Stacy called out one hand outstretched pushing his shoulder, the other treading water as they whisked by helpless onlookers standing on walkways and bridges above them. A third ring, louder now.

"Stan! Answer the phone!" She kicked away from him into the arms of a man groping her in obvious lust, both of them laughing.

"Aren't you going to answer the phone?"

The building dissolved. Stan felt thumping on his back and heard the fourth ring, now in the darkness of his bedroom. His hand flailed, knocking a bible on the floor as well as a pager before it found the phone.

"Hello?" He managed a barely audible croak.

"Dr. Blackstone, this is the answering service. I have a call for you, can you take it?" "What?"

"The ICU at Olympus is on the phone. Can you take the call?"

No answer.

"Dr. Blackstone, are you awake?"

"Yeah," he lied.

"I'm putting the call through now."

"Hello, Dr. Blackstone?"

"Yeah. I'm here."

"This is Mandy in the cardiac ICU taking care of Mrs. Thompson. Her cardiac output is staying under two liters a minute on dobutamine, levophed and milrinone. Dr. Malloy thought I should let you know in case you wanted to put the balloon pump in sooner."

Large red numbers, four, three and seven, levitated above him on the bedside table.

"Is it 4:30?"

"It is."

"I'll put it in at seven."

"That's right at shift change. Could you do it before?"

"Sure. 6:50."

There was a sigh on the other end of the line. "You heard me say she's not doing well?"

"I'm not hearing impaired." Blackstone rested his head on the pillow, enjoying his wit. He took pride in his steep resistance to coming in at night and his reliance on faith to preserve his patients until his mind was fresh. His tired mind, however, drifted and he was once again floating down a steaming river into an ominous, dark future.

"Her lactic acid is up and her pH is 7.29. Are you sure you want to wait?"

No answer.

"Dr. Blackstone?"

The line was open and silent. Maybe a snore? The information she delivered indicated Sarah was in shock, her heart was not pumping enough blood to deliver oxygen to many of the cells in the body. Without oxygen, metabolism changed to anaerobic, producing lactic acid. She slammed the phone down. In her anger she decided to write him up, once again, in an incident report.

At 7:30 Sunday morning, Blackstone entered the cardiac catheterization lab where he would insert of a long balloon through the femoral artery and under fluoroscopy position it in the segment of the aorta that leads from the top of the chest to the upper abdomen. There it would inflate when the heart is filling and deflate as the heart pumps augmenting her blood pressure and improving cardiac output. The procedure did not take long and was not complex. Half an hour later, Sarah was attached to the balloon console, one more machine keeping her alive.

Blackstone made a call to the Wasatch clinic and spoke with a junior cardiologist, a transplant "fellow" who was making rounds there. They had a bed available and would be happy to accept her in transfer. He arranged a helicopter ambulance and spoke with a heart surgeon.

After Blackstone finished his phone calls and dictation of the procedure he went to the ICU. Sarah's blood pressure was a little higher and her cardiac output up to two point four liters per minute. This was still well below normal but enough, he hoped. A young round-headed girl ran into the ICU as the doors burst open, followed by the parents of his patient.

"Dr. Blackstone!" Myra called out as she wheezed from effort.

He waved them to the doorway of Sarah's room.

"How is Sarah?"

"She had a bad night. Her condition deteriorated despite our best efforts. I had to put a balloon pump in her."

"Maybe changing her treatment was a bad idea," Ed said.

"I saved her life. Dr. Harrison waited too long, did nothing," Dr. Blackstone replied. "I thought this would happen, which is why I transferred her to the ICU."

Amy was in the room, standing with four fingers in her mouth, lip quivering, eyebrows angling in and up, water gathering over her blue eyes, slipping down her face, one cheek at a time. Two nurses worked on the person that lay in the bed that belonged to her mother.

"Oh, God. Oh, dear God." Myra wrung her hands and swayed. "What are you going to do now?"

"I am going to transfer her to the heart failure center. I spoke with a couple of the doctors that have agreed to take care of her. A helicopter is on the way."

"Dr. Harrison warned us that might be needed," Ed said.

"We never even met the man, Ed," Myra said. "How do you know that?"

"Sarah mentioned it."

"I didn't hear it. She thought she was just going to get better."

"Wishful thinking never cured anyone," Blackstone said. "She will probably go on the urgent transplant list. They might put her on an artificial heart or another machine, a ventricular assist device called a VAD."

"Will that save her life?" Myra asked.

"Probably."

Ed went in the room and held Amy's tiny hand, then took a knee next to her.

"Where Mommy?"

"She's in the bed. She got very sick and these nurses and machines are working hard to make her better."

"Can I see?"

He lifted her up and brought her closer. Sarah's eyes were taped shut. A yellow tube was taped to her nose, running into a nostril. A finger-sized plastic pipe, secured with white tape, disappeared into her mouth. Blood-tinged saliva oozed from the corner of her mouth. Sight and the assortment of odors brought his morning coffee back into his mouth.

"Are you sure you want her to remember this?" O'Toole asked Ed.

"Probably not."

"You should get a nice picture of her from home and let her look at that instead of this," she recommended. "She'll have nightmares for years."

Ed hugged Amy, twisted her head away where it had been transfixed. She struggled to see. "You don't want to see your mommy like, this, sugar plum."

She looked him straight in the eye. He stood, took her hand and together they walked away.

"Ed, what are you doing?"

"She shouldn't see her mom like that."

"Nonsense."

"We'll argue about this later." He left for the waiting room, fighting Amy's persistent squirm.

"Humph." She entered the room.

Slowly waddling forward, the image of her baby came into focus. Stunned, horrified by the mosaic of technology, biology, smells, sounds, engineering, nurses, metal, glass, plastic and fabric filled by the grout of impending loss and cemented to the receding life of her only daughter, her jaw shuddered in horror before she collapsed.

Stan Blackstone was sitting in church, cradling his sleeping one-year-old daughter when the helicopter lifted off with Sarah Thompson.

A little after 10:00 in the evening he was back in the hospital with a new patient when Emil Sarfatian, a heart surgeon, called him.

"We just finished putting a VAD in Mrs. Thompson," he explained in an accent unfamiliar to Blackstone. "Her pressure was in the toilet for quite a while. I hope she's okay. Next time, you should think about transfer a little sooner."

"I'm just covering for one of my partners. I had little choice in the matter."

"Ward heard about her last Thursday. If she came on Friday or Saturday, it would have been a lot easier on everyone. We've had a rough time keeping her alive."

"We all had a rough time," Stan said.

"I'm afraid she might not wake up."

"Thanks for the follow-up. Have a blessed day." Blackstone hung up without waiting for a reply. *She'll be in a better place*, he thought until he realized Harrison had, once again, put him in a bad position, making him look bad to the doctors at Wasatch.

He tried not to hate Harrison. It was a mortal trial for his soul to "love thine enemy" when it came to his soon-to-be ex-partner. He could not help but nurture the familiar litany of complaints he had nurtured over the years. Harrison's pride, gluttony, lust, greed and other vices had damaged him. He had stolen his earnings for years, had treated him unfairly with night and weekend call. It would be so nice to get even. "Vengeance is mine, saith the Lord." If Sally died he could perhaps nudge the retribution along. Cheryl ... Shauna ... or whatever her blessed name was.

Blackstone turned his attention back to the eighty-eight-year-old who had a heart attack several days before, but delayed coming in until his family visited late Sunday afternoon. It made no eternal sense that his presence was needed at this late hour. He should have stayed home, phoned in orders and looked at the patient in the morning. But, no, that was not allowed because Harrison that had made the rule that patients get seen when admitted, not the next day. What a stupid use of his time.

Chapter 15

Around noon on Monday Dr. Bill Ward stopped Dr. Sarfatian for a short chat in the thoracic ICU after the neurologist left Sarah Thompson's room. "When Harrison talked to me about her, he said she had been stable the whole week. Perhaps I should have told him to send her then."

"Maybe but she didn't go south until Saturday," Sarfatian explained. "She should have been transferred then."

"Are you going to tell Blackstone that?"

"I don't know. I've got to be nice so he'll send stuff here and not to the competition."

Sarfatian hesitated as he considered his words, then punched in the numbers for the required phone call.

"Dr. Blackstone." There was a sound of chewing on the speakerphone.

"This is Emil, from the University. Is this a good time to talk?"

"I'm just eating lunch packed by my lovely wife. Go ahead."

"I'm here with Dr. Ward. We thought I should let you know what's going on with Thompson. She hasn't woken up. EEG this morning looks bad."

"This is Harrison's fault. He mistreated her for a week."

"Like I said last night, she had almost no blood pressure for quite a long time. I think that killed her squash."

They heard chewing.

"The neurologist said he wants to repeat another EEG tomorrow before we pull the plug."

"Well, she'll be in a better place," Blackstone stated with certainty and conviction. "Harrison mistreated her for a week. I did everything I could and so did you. Our hands are clean."

Sarfatian furrowed his brow.

Ward recoiled. "It would've nice if you had transferred her a day or two earlier," Ward said after a pause.

"Sheila was doomed, given the first week of her care."

Both of them raised eyebrows.

"Her name is Sarah." Ward shook his head.

"My resident or I will call you when we have new information," Sarfatian said.

"Let Harrison know. My work with her is done." Blackstone hung up.

Sarfatian turned to Ward. "And I thought we were dysfunctional."

Blackstone gobbled the last remaining bites of his lunch and washed it down with his bottled tea. He charged out of his office and down a few doors. He found Malouf and Pierce meeting with the administrator, Charla and barged in.

"Harrison just killed a thirty-year-old wife and mother. Just basically an assassination."

No one responded, to Blackstone's surprise. "He should be fired for cause. This is a travesty."

"Write it up," Malouf said. "We'll deal with it in conference. We're in the middle of...."

"It is my mission to destroy this man," Stan declared. "I will shred his license and expose his malfeasance, destroy his reputation and make it so he'll never work as a cardiologist again. I'm so sick and tired of this whole mess!"

"Stan, we're together on that," Pierce said. "But we're in a meeting. Now is not a good time." Pierce stood as if to shoo him out.

"I'm not going to stop with just getting him out of the practice. I want his license. I want him in poverty and unemployable."

"We're busy here, Stan," Malouf said.

Stan felt disrespected as he backed out, punctuated by the forceful closure of the door. As soon as he got into his room he picked up his tiny recorder and began dictating an angry tale of how Harrison had utterly failed this patient and abandoned her, dumping her on him. Despite his Herculean efforts, he had been unable to turn the tide of her slide, as he liked to say.

Early Tuesday afternoon in a small conference room near the Thoracic ICU Dr. Sarfatian, together with his chief thoracic surgery resident, a cardiology heart failure "fellow" and a neurology resident, met with Myra and Ed Szabo. It had been a long, slow journey from the front door for Ed. Myra kept stopping for air then griping about the distance and the heat and the smell and the tattoos and piercings and many other things as she gasped along her way.

The neurologist greeted them in a subtle accent and shook their hands warmly. He talked. The EEG and the examination showed she was brain dead without a chance of recovery. Her driver's license indicated she was an organ donor. Other voices spoke, a chaplain, a social worker, Dr. Sarfatian. They were kind but in no doubt.

Ed surveyed the scene through bloodshot eyes, his senses keen, his mind racing to keep up with the verbal barrage. The building did not smell of ether and alcohol as they did when he was young. There were no instruments soaking in stainless steel trays. Now it seemed almost everything was disposable, single use, not reused. But they were asking if they could recycle parts of his daughter.

The nurses no longer wore starched, clean uniforms, white caps and shoes. Sarah's nurse was a man with a soul-patch, a gold ring in his right ear. A black rose was tattooed on his forearm. It was nothing like when Sarah was born in the Marchetti wing of what was then Waters of Bethesda Hospital, built with granite, maple and plaster on lathe and filled with female nurses in starched white uniforms. In all the progress leading to this bleakest of days they were preparing her desecration, a "harvest," as they said, of her corneas, skin, bone, liver and kidneys. It was her wish, they stated without ever knowing her, hearing her laugh, holding her when she cried, listening to her day, her challenges, her conflicts her idle chatter. They knew because of two words printed on a government issued card in her wallet. They knew everything and nothing.

A chaplain placed his hand on Myra's shoulder. He wore an open shirt and wrinkled Dockers pants under a too-small white pharmacist jacket. Doc Martin sandals buckled over his argyle socks. He had a ruddy, plump face, a happy smile and red hair gone white. The doctors were young, astute overachievers, talking without feelings, bruises or scars.

Myra wobbled in the chair, stunned with grief. Ed rested his hand on her shoulder.

"Yes," he said.

The room emptied.

He checked the time, needing to return to work. He had given his notice for retirement in June. With the loss of Sarah's donation to their income, he would rescind it. As of today he could no longer afford to stop working. His insurance would be needed to support Amy.

Sarah was declared dead on Tuesday afternoon but was kept biologically functional as the organ procurement company, ReSorce, assumed financial responsibility for her care as they matched recipients for her parts that were functional. The Szabos along with Amy would see her two days later in the mortuary.

Chapter 16

October 2005

The pencil-thin mustache was still there but Hugh Harrison's hair was now trimmed, crisp and clean. His sideburns had been severed as was his relationship with Ashleigh. The only good thing about that was the absence of boy noise, arguments, juvenile television, video games and potty humor. Sipping amber liquid under melting ice cubes, he missed the conversations of things outside medicine and Ashleigh's refreshing perspectives of events, life, cause-and-effect and humanity, which she loved to analyze. He wanted to hear about the unruly girls and the gawky boys and the process of growing up. He longed for the smell of her straight brown hair, the feel of her long feet, legs and fingers. The absence of conversation sucked life from the room no longer in chaos with extra furniture, clothing, toys and cat. Order was restored. His journals and a few of her magazines lay in two neat stacks. Pillows were fluffed and positioned artistically on the sofa, recently cleaned.

Ashe's soft faux fur rug still lay before the hearth where they had explored, explained, examined, exorcised and exulted. It reminded him of the moment she told him she was leaving.

She began with his words. "As you say, Hugh, it's impossible to be perfectly honest and perfectly kind." She chose neither that evening, speaking circumspect half-truths, trying not to end things with a fight. She gave him and her students truth without quarter or hostility. He loved her for that and a thousand other reasons. How he felt was irrelevant, at this point. He was an inadequate, unsatisfactory mate. He hoped the reasons she gave would become understandable with time. But her words confused him and tonight, again, he relied on Scotch to make clear their meaning. It was invariably a poor solution and he knew it.

He carried the tumbler into the office where it found a coaster, still damp from earlier in the morning. A file drawer extended open six inches from the desk where colored tabs organized his battles.

Yellow marked malpractice papers for Thompson and Szabo versus Wren, Barton, Blackstone, Harrison, Malloy, Two Rivers Internal Medicine, Chandler Cardiovascular Clinic, OCHA Medical Center and its owner, Auspicious Healthcare. Tomorrow was the first major skirmish, his deposition. Hundreds of pages of medical records were punched and tabbed in two thick binders in the birch hutch behind his desk.

Blue indicated his breach of contract suit against Chandler Cardiovascular and their countersuit against him. They had kept hundreds of thousands of dollars of his money, his deferred compensation, stock purchase and his accounts receivable, claiming he had breached his contract, to which he had assiduously strived to comply. It was maddening.

The files with red were collections of information about the actions of OCHA and his former group that contributed to the failure of Saint Lucius Medical Center. When the hospital closed its doors after less than a year of operation one month ago, he began collecting papers and writing his recollections.

He sighed at the prospect of preparing for the deposition in the morning. He knocked back the last swallow and decided he couldn't face going over the medical records again. He picked up an international intrigue novel and settled into a recliner. Two bulging black loose-leaf books with medical records waited on the adjacent table.

CHAPTER 17

Early Monday morning Harrison tamped down his headache with caffeine and acetaminophen as he quickly saw his few hospitalized patients that remained from his weekend off duty. He then hurried downtown to the law office of Hundley Hart.

He took an elevator to the twelfth floor. He took a lap around the corridor until he found a door of security glass displaying Suite 1209, Hundley Hart. The smell of cinnamon and ginger hit as he entered. His attorney, Monica Jessop, appointed by his malpractice company, sat in the waiting room. She was in her early forties, in heels a little taller than her client and wore a dark blue suit, a beige blouse open at the neck framing a textured pewter cross. She appeared fit. Her straight light brown hair hung to her shoulders.

She had instructed him to wear a suit, which he had to purchase. She offered her hand and they shook.

"I'm glad you're a little early, Dr. Harrison," she began. "I wanted to go over one more," she paused looking for the right word, "notion with you before we start."

"What might that be?"

"First off, did you sleep well?"

"Well enough."

She studied him closely. "You lie poorly, Doctor."

He said nothing.

"One thing that Dennis may do is try to get you to blame Dr. Blackstone or someone else. You and Dr. Blackstone have the same malpractice carrier and their interest is to protect both of you and to keep the total financial expenditures as low as possible. If Dennis asks questions about the care of Dr. Blackstone I will object and instruct you not to answer."

"His approach was radically different than mine," Harrison said, rubbing his forehead. "Only an idiot would fail to pursue that."

"You should explain your actions only, without blaming Blackstone or anyone else," she said. "You're not an expert witness in this case. Don't offer medical opinions, just statements about what you did."

"Are you representing me or the insurance company? After all, they are the ones paying you." He regretted challenging her but it just came out before he had a chance to fetch it back.

"I represent you but I need to keep their situation in mind."

She looked at her small watch and started moving back to the law office, motioning Dr. Harrison to follow. "If you need to think or get tired, tell me and we'll take a break."

A pudgy man in a rumpled tweed suit rounded the corner and approached, scratching his nose with one hand while the other toted a leather briefcase.

Monica stopped. "Hi, Stan," she said. "I thought you might show up for this."

"Hello, Monica."

"Dr. Harrison, this is Stan Henriod, attorney for both Dr. Blackstone and

Chandler Cardiovascular. He's going to listen in. The hospital's defense attorney should show up as well."

They shook hands. "A Stan defending a Stan. Could get confusing."

"I'm Stanley and he is Stanton. I'm not confused."

"Are you two from the same firm?" Hugh asked.

"Hunter Hinkley. Yep." Henriod was fair with freckled, ruddy cheeks, looking like a Scot with an addiction to pastry.

They entered Hart's office. Harrison noticed the oriental rug, an inlaid floor, expensive furniture and original art. A lot of money had gone into this room from doctors Hart had successfully extorted or destroyed. A candle flickered on the empty receptionist's desk filling the room with a dark floral scent.

They sat for less than a minute before the door opened. A large man with gray hair, reading glasses halfway down his nose, a light blue shirt with cuffs rolled up his burly forearms, smiled and spoke. "Hi, Monica, Stan. This must be Dr. Harrison?"

"Yes."

"Dennis Hart," he said, extending a thick hand. "Come in. The court reporter and videographer are both here and ready to go."

"Videographer?" Monica asked.

"We video all our depositions."

"That was not in the summons," she argued.

The conflict had begun.

"Doctor, before we get into the details of your treatment of the deceased, I noticed that your approach to her management was different than that of your partner, Dr. Blackstone. Why is that?"

"Dr. Blackstone never explained his decisions to me." Harrison noticed his attorney perk up.

"Did you explain your treatment plan to him when you signed out?"

"Yes."

"Do you recall what you said to him?"

"I don't have an independent recollection of our conversation." He had that line memorized.

"So, how do you know you explained your management?"

"We all give a list of names and locations with a brief sketch of the problems to the on call guy along with test results pending and a general plan. It's routine. I vaguely remember having a conversation with Stan but now, a year and a half later, I don't recall exactly what was said."

"Fair enough. Do you remember generally what you said?"

"As I said, I don't remember the details."

"A young mother getting progressively worse with a life-threatening disease and you do not recall even generally what you told Dr. Blackstone to do?"

"I conveyed that I had been taking a conservative approach and that Dr. Ward was willing to accept her in transfer if she deteriorated."

"You did not refer her for a transplant, did you?"

"Correct."

"Why not?"

"Her clinical condition meaning her weight, blood pressure, heart rate and symptoms were stable. Her ejection fraction was falling but we were watching that frequently. It was not severely impaired when I left."

"Is it true that heart transplantation is the only cure for this condition?"

"The vast majority of people with myocarditis get better on their own. For the few with progressive disease, transplant is the only effective solution."

"You are not a specialist in heart failure, are you?"

"Not beyond being a cardiologist."

"Does it not seem appropriate to refer a young mother to the highest level of care possible for what proved to be a fatal condition?"

"The level of care at Olympus was appropriate for the majority of patients with myocarditis."

"But not for Mrs. Thompson, correct?"

"In retrospect and after the pathology was known, that is correct."

"Did you consider that she might have a more serious type of disease?"

"That's why I talked with Dr. Ward about her before I left town."

"Would her life have been saved had you transferred her that Friday?"

"I object," Jessop said. "Calls for speculation. I'm instructing my client not to answer."

Harrison could not hold back. "On Friday it was not clear that her condition was going to be fatal. Moreover, heart failure patients did better at OCHA than at Wasatch based on published outcome data. Unless she needed a procedure we could not provide, I saw no benefit in transferring her."

Hart scratched his scalp and removed his reading glasses. "Where did you come up with that?"

"A website that reports outcomes based on public data."

"I find that hard to believe," Hart reacted, then waited for a response.

Harrison remained quiet.

"Let's take a break," Hart said.

The red camera light went off, the reporter lifted his hands from the small black box he used for stenography.

"Monica," Hart said, "could you get me the web address Dr. Harrison referred to?"

She gave him a name as everyone but one reporter exited the room. Harrison and Jessop conferred in a small office nearby. "You're doing great. That was a good answer to the last question. I didn't know that."

"I found the site yesterday. I didn't know it at the time."

When they came back there was more small talk as if Hart, Henriod and Jessop were friends. The session reconvened.

"Doctor, do you agree with how Dr. Blackstone managed your patient?"

"I object," Monica asserted. "Irrelevant. Dr. Harrison is here with respect to his actions, not as an expert witness."

"Objection noted," Hart said. "I'm not asking for an expert opinion, just whether these two doctors were in agreement. Please answer the question, Doctor."

"I am instructing my client not to answer."

"Well, Doctor?"

"Don't answer," Monica said.

Harrison wanted to answer. He thought the actions of his former partner hastened the demise of the young woman. Jessop and Henriod whispered as he made a decision. Sarah should have survived long enough to get appropriate treatment and would have, Harrison was certain, if he had not left her in the hands of Stan Blackstone. "I'm going to comply with the advice of counsel," was a leap of faith made against his instinct of self-preservation and desire to disparage his former partner.

The rest of the day was spent going over his notes, orders and the rationale behind each. Details were teased out of the brevity used in medical records. Late in the afternoon Hart changed direction.

"You left Chandler Cardiovascular Clinic shortly after Ms. Thompson died, did you not?"

"A few months later."

"Were you not the cardiologist that built the group and managed it for years?"

"Not completely. Nigel Sampson and I joined Randy Chandler's existing practice and after Chandler died, I ran it for five or six years."

"Why did you leave?"

"Objection. Relevance."

"The answer addresses the relationship between the defendants," Hart argued. "The judge will rule on your objection later. Doctor, please answer the question."

Jessop nodded.

Harrison answered, "The values of the newer partners were too much of a departure from the beginning."

Hart paused as he scribbled on his yellow notepad, taking a few additional seconds with his eyes screwed shut in apparent thought.

"Values? Did Chandler Cardiovascular have a formal statement of its vision and values?"

"Vision, yes. Values no."

"Can you describe one value and how it changed so much that you felt compelled to leave the group you built?"

"My position has always been that we take care of the patient first in the best way possible. After that, we work on how to optimize our income. By the time I left, this was reversed, maximizing income through a proliferation of procedures."

"Can you be specific, Doctor?"

Harrison took a deep breath, expanding a moment to figure out where to begin to skewer, under oath, his former colleagues. So many choices, he thought. The cardiac catheterization lab issues with hundreds angioplasties done unnecessarily on minor blockages and pacemakers implanted for benign conditions. Then there were the thousands of stress tests done to fill patients or their doctors with a false sense of security without having any positive impact on their health and the echocardiograms done every three or six months on unsuspecting souls with mitral valve prolapse that was typically imaginary at worst and benign at best and the echoes for other trivial reasons as well. These filled the coffers of both his former practice and an unknown number of similar practices all over the country.

"I'm instructing my client not to answer," Monica said. "This is completely irrelevant."

"I see," Hart said, squinting.

Harrison ached to answer, to put the practices on record under oath. Instead he followed advice not to offer any information and to answer questions as briefly as possible. He took a deep breath and leaned back.

Hart soon ended the deposition with the proviso that he could reopen it later and take one more bite of the apple, in lawyer lingo.

CHAPTER 18

Ed Szabo wedged his dark blue Toyota Camry into the small parking lot and playground of Winkler School a little after 4:30, between large SUVs of other parents or guardians who were picking up kids. Amy, barely eleven years old, looked through the wire reinforced glass pane in the door as her grandfather got out of the car in blazing sunshine and started walking in her direction. A young teacher's aide gave her permission to leave. She burst out of the door and clumsily hugged Ed, her daily ritual. As usual, he almost fell over. Amy was growing both in height and girth. Ed was shrinking, more gaunt and gray. This was the best moment of his day, the few minutes he spent with this little girl. She filled a bit of the void that had begun a year and a half earlier.

"Hi, Gwamps," she said as she release her grip around his arms and chest.

"It's so good to see you, Punkin'." He took her hand as they walked to the car. He put her backpack in the back seat and helped her with the seatbelt. "What did you do in school today, sweetie?"

"Painted. We painted bowls."

"Were they clay bowls?"

"Just bowls."

She made a cupping shape with her short-fingered hands. A small lump grew deep in his throat as he remembered Sarah working with clay. One of her glazed and fired figures, a Kokopelli, dangled from a hemp twine around the rearview mirror.

"Will you bring the bowl home?"

"I think."

And therefore she is, Ed ruminated, knuckling a burning away from his pink lid, the only color on his face. He glanced at her then back at the road.

Sensing his look, she turned with a smile. "I missed you, Gwamps."

"And I missed you."

It was Monday and Doug made it a point to have Amy spend weekends with him. It worried Ed because Doug was irresponsible but motivated to have the weekends with his daughter in hope of a bigger payout from the malpractice suit.

When they arrived home, Myra sat on the covered porch in their home built over eighty years earlier. A huge elm arched over much of the yard, leaves bright yellow. Pyracanthas bordered the house. The driveway was gravel and ended in a separate old wooden garage. Both structures needed paint. Rather than go in the back door, they walked around to the front. The walkway was uneven. Amy stepped playfully around the dips and bumps.

Myra rocked with a red-and-white afghan draped over her knees, growing as she worked two long needles and skeins of wool yarn. A tall iced tea sweated on a wicker table nearby. Seven worn wooden steps led to the porch. Amy put her right foot up on the first step, then her left, climbing one step at a time. Ed noticed she put her right hand on her rump as she climbed.

Amy did not hug Myra but went inside the house.

Ed leaned the pink backpack against the rail posts, knocking off flecks of peeling paint. "What's up?"

Myra did not look up from her handwork. "I'm making good progress on this throw."

He knew it had not grown much since yesterday or last week. She spent most of her day doing something other than knitting, probably watching television. She had gained a lot of weight in the last eighteen months. Her fingers were nicked from blood sugar tests she did once or twice a day, more than she wanted and less than what she should have been doing. A quarter of an inch of gray showed at the base of her hair. She pursed her lips to exhale.

"How are you feeling?"

"This damn arthritis is killing me," she replied, extending her two little fingers with knobby joints.

"The medicine doesn't help?"

"I take so many pills already. I don't want any more. We go broke just buying the prescriptions." She scowled as a couple of kids rolled past the house in the street on skateboards, faces screwed tight, intent. "How does your boss feel about you leaving early to pick up Amy?"

"He likes me coming in early, so it works out well, so he says."

"I hope so. I don't want you losing your job."

"Do you have anything planned for dinner?"

"No."

"Is it okay if I fix some pasta?"

"No tomato in the sauce, Ed."

He picked up the pack and went into the house. Amy was not in the front room or kitchen. He looked for her in the bedrooms, bathrooms and closets. The attic was locked. He didn't see her in the backyard so he climbed down the steep steps into the cellar. A single bulb burned from the ceiling. Amy pointed at the octopus of aluminum ducts as she walked along underneath each, mumbling. Beyond her was a black iron cover on the old fuel chute. He had removed the wooden bin himself about the time he moved in. Now, a high-efficiency natural gas furnace took up a small fraction of the space of the original but much of the ductwork remained. The room would forever smell of coal.

"What are you doing down here, Amy?"

"Pipes," she said as she traced routes. "Big pipes."

"Do you know what the pipes are for?"

"No."

He had explained this a dozen times in the past. He decided not to repeat it now. "They are pretty," he said.

She raised a hand, splayed her fingers mimicking the configuration and twirled. Then she fell. The challenge of keeping balance and pointing up was too much. *Sad for an eleven-year-old,* Ed thought as he started forward then stopped, knowing she needed to get up and take care of herself. She did not cry, just got up and brushed off the dust and cobwebs.

"What do you want for dinner, Amy?"

"Mac and cheese," she said. That was her typical response.

"Can you help me fix dinner?"

She came to where he stood, took his hand and pulled him to the stairs. Climbing in front of him, she put a hand on her butt again.

When they got into the kitchen, Ed asked, "Do you have a hurt on your bottom?"

"Tat," she said.

"What?" He didn't understand.

"Tat."

"Would you show me?"

She pulled her pants down enough so he could see a colorful tattoo on her rump with a little crusting of serum.

"When did you get this?"

She moved her fingers over the area. "Tat. Fluff-fly."

Butterfly, Ed understood. "Did you want that?"

"Yes."

"Did it hurt?"

"Yes, but it was Daddy happy."

It occurred to Ed that Amy's language skill had perhaps regressed since Sarah's death. He committed to work on it.

"Let's get cooking," he said.

About nine-thirty the phone rang. Ed answered.

"How's Amy?"

"She's fine, Doug."

Ed put the phone on speaker. Myra muted the television.

"No problems?"

"I see she has a tattoo. What's that all about?"

"She wanted it, so—"

"She has a what?" Myra cackled.

Ed shook his head in disgust.

"You got a problem with that, Ed?"

"I don't like it."

"She's not your daughter. She asked for it and I got it for her, like a good dad." He loomed over his ex-father-in-law. "Anyways," Doug softened, "thanks for picking her up after school. I'll have this pub job for another month or two until ski season starts."

"I think it's good for her to spend some time with us," Ed opined. "I'd like her to come here in the winter as well."

"We'll see. That might work out because the chick I'm seeing now doesn't really like kids, particularly if they are, uh, different. But, who knows if she'll still around in a month?"

"I can only imagine what effect the parade of sluts through your bedroom has on Amy," Myra said.

"They're not sluts and they've been nice to her. Did Hart talk to you today?" Doug asked.

"Yeah," Myra said. "Did you call you?"

"Not at work and my cell isn't working. What did he say?"

"He seemed pleased with the day. He'll depose Dr. Blackstone tomorrow and the internists later this week. He's spending the entire week on this case."

"Does he smell money?"

"I hope he rips those bastards for every stinking penny," Myra said.

"I'm not sure he's mean enough," Doug said. "We'll see how he does for a while. Somebody needs to teach those privileged jackasses a lesson. It might as well be us." A woman's voice sounded in the background. "Gotta get off this phone," he said and hung up.

"The gift that keeps on giving," Ed mumbled.

"What was that, Ed?"

"I was just thinking that some of our mistakes are with us for life."

"That's why I knit."

Those were the errors she could undo, Ed went to the bedroom, peaking in at Amy sleeping as he passed her room. He closed the door and opened *Fountainhead* somewhere around page six hundred.

"It was good that we couldn't meet a week ago," Malouf said, sitting forward at the head of the corporate table. "It gave Carla time to finish the third quarter financials."

About a dozen cardiologists were already leafing through the several pages of figures inside the Chandler Cardiovascular Clinic boardroom Monday evening.

"I think you'll agree they look good."

"No, they look great," Pierce gurgled. "That's going to give us a rather large third-quarter bonus this month."

"That is one hell of a lot of money," said Nigel Sampson in utter surprise.

"Everything other than the cath lab has been stable financially, with a little extra growth in the echo and nuclear imaging again," observed Malouf. "But the biggest increase is the cath lab because the contract has been in place for over a year and cash flow has doubled our profit."

Carla, a stocky woman with a masculine face, handed each physician a windowed envelope containing a bonus check as Sarisha continued. "As usual, we are paying out eighty percent of the bonus today and will pay out the complete amount at the end of the year."

Stanton Blackstone was among the first to rip open the gift. His jaw fell initially then his mouth phased into a smile. His year-to-date income was now well over $500,000. He looked and pointed up, mouthing, "Thank you, God."

"This is too much," said Chimwuanya Obi-Poku in his lilting Sub-Saharan accent.

"This is your first bonus, Jim," Malouf said. "It is the largest we have ever had by far. We deducted some of the amount you are paying for stock to become an owner and it's still a lot of money. Aren't you glad you joined?"

"Very happy," he said with a large, toothy smile.

"Sarisha," Dr. Pierce said, "you're doing great as the managing physician." He started to applaud and was immediately joined by everyone.

After a couple of courtesy claps, Sampson ran a hand across his short blond hair, trying to hide his aversion. While he and Harrison had many deep differences, they had a couple of traits and values in common. He agreed with him that the focus of the practice had changed. He kept his dissatisfaction hidden as well as his new job offer from Arizona. His resignation letter was ready to be printed, reserved until he and his wife agreed on the relocation.

A few minutes later Jonathan Gullimore, who had been sitting quietly against the outside wall, stood to address the group. "Dr. Malouf asked me to update you about the legal status of the suit and countersuit with Hugh Harrison." He adjusted his tie. His suitcoat was draped around the back of his chair. "I will be deposing him on Thursday. I picked this week because he was deposed today on a malpractice matter and should be emotionally off his peak."

"How much is he asking for?" Ted Hatcher asked.

"A total of $1.7 million."

Sampson looked at the financial sheet and saw the total profit to be shared between the fourteen cardiologists approached three million dollars for one quarter. Half of that would pay Harrison about what he was asking and still leave everyone with a generous bonus. He and everyone in the room had benefitted richly from Harrison's work although the recent boost was from Malouf's lab contract. He bit his tongue and rubbed his crew cut once again, feeling guilt.

"He's a greedy mother," Hatcher said.

"Did you project our legal fees will be about two hundred thousand?" Montgomery Pierce.

"Probably more, up to five hundred if we don't go to trial. It depends greatly on how long this takes. We can wage a slow war of attrition and exhaust him of money and heart."

"We have a lot of assets to use in this case," Malouf said. "I think it is critical that we send a message that you don't mess with us. What it may cost us this time, we may save in the future." This was not a just a defense against Hugh Harrison only; it was a warning for everyone at the table.

"Just how solid is the case?" Sampson asked.

"Rock," the attorney replied.

"It seems like not a good way to part with a senior founder."

"Like you," Malouf said curtly.

Sampson felt the tension rise as he waited to answer with equanimity. "For example," was his response.

"You can't have senior people leaving. You all went on the hook for a loan to expand the practice including the cath lab venture," Gullimore said. "Leaving that debt burden to junior associates would potentially be devastating. The contract puts everyone on the hook financially."

"Debatable," said Sampson. "You could pay off the loan with less than half of this quarter's bonus, plus pay him a million and everyone still has a good bonus and goodwill."

This was met with grating silence.

"What about our countersuit?" Malouf asked.

"After he is deposed on Thursday, I hope to have enough to seek summary judgment to dismiss his claim and grant ours. His action is frivolous and malicious and you should be awarded all your legal fees and some punitive damages."

"Yeah," Blackstone cheered.

"Oh, let it alone," Obi-Poku whispered with a disappointed frown.

Afterward Sampson drove to the Country Club driving range and blasted a bucket of balls before closing. He made a call to the hospital in Cottonwood Arizona as he drove home to his one-acre wooded lot that backed onto a small stream. Tonight he had to make his wife see that he needed to leave.

CHAPTER 20

Leo Damjanovich was with a firm of about twenty other attorneys, Dingle & Damjanovich, which he started thirty-five years earlier. He had a long face, round glasses perched on a beak of a nose and a baritone voice. "Gullimore is going to make a big deal out of the wording of the agreement."

"As attorneys do," Harrison said.

"For today, remember you should not offer information. Just say yea or nay where possible. Nothing said here will help your cause. You can either damage it or not, preferably not."

"Understood."

They entered a tall building and within minutes were sitting at a conference table in Gullimore's office. A woman about thirty swore Harrison to tell the truth then started both her tape recorder and stenographer's machine to record the encounter. An hour and a half later the little ground that had been covered was done so meticulously. They took a break.

"It looks like his strategy is to tire you out with minutia then hit with the hard questions later," Leo observed before they reentered the room.

"Billable hours. It's how you make money."

No response as they walked in. The court reporter sipped from a bottle of water.

"Hi, Sarisha," Harrison said.

Malouf had joined and sat against the wall away from the long table.

"Hugh," she said and nodded, game-faced.

If I bought her for her worth and sold her for what she thought she was worth, I'd drop this suit, money ahead, Harrison thought.

Gullimore introduced Hugh's employment agreement as exhibit four, his deferred compensation agreement as exhibit five and the stock buy-sell agreement as exhibit six. Each of these documents was between fifteen and forty pages in length, mostly comprised of boilerplate verbiage with some specifics pertinent to Chandler Cardiovascular. He then spent endless hours dissecting the arcane and tedious language

Late in the afternoon the court reporter indicated her eight hours was up. Gullimore was not done. He requested a continuance of the deposition to be arranged at a future date.

Shortly after the deposition ended Don Zone, Jennifer Hayes and Chad Mixon sat around the end of the conference table in OCHA boardroom. An open bottle of 1997 Silver Oak Cabernet stood sentry amidst papers strewn about in random organization. Mixon, troubled, looked out the window as Hayes sipped and Zone swirled glasses of wine. He was deathly afraid of going to jail for what they, he had done. Inside his coat a small Dictaphone recorder was on. He needed to get some defense in case the Feds came knocking.

"Congratulations on killing Saint Lucius," Zone said, raising his glass.

They all clinked and sipped.

"I hope there's no eternal retribution for defeating nuns," Mixon said.

"Today a *For Sale* banner went up on the side of the building. Other than destroying competition, I am most pleased that we had such good teamwork and strategy. Jennifer, you had great foresight when you crafted the managed care contracts. That was huge, the foundation of success."

"It was a gamble," she admitted. "A speed bump that would use up a competitor's money and time during a startup when they could least afford it."

Zone continued. "You kept Grant Orthopaedics and Chandler Cardiovascular from going there. That nailed the place shut. What a great move."

"It was expensive," Chad interjected.

"Not as bad as losing revenue to a competing hospital," Hayes said.

"Our payments to Chandler are huge," Chad pointed out.

"Again, in the big picture, a small price to pay." Hayes looked at him like he was an idiot.

"Does it bother you that it might be viewed as fraud?" Mixon squirmed.

"We've been over this before, Chad," Don chastised. "It is not illegal. It's outsourcing."

"For a service we already offered. Then there's the doing a procedure in their lab and billing it as if it were done here. It looks questionable." Mixon broke out in a sweat every time they discussed the issue.

"Legal gave us the green light," Zone said. "Relax. Their necks are on the line on this one."

"It amounts to—"

A deep thump shook the room, Zones List on the table. "I don't want to hear any more whining! Chad, this is how you get a win. We fought hard against Saint's and shut 'em down. Chandler is in our pocket and the big boys in corporate are happy."

Chad lowered his eyes. He said no more. He wanted to check his recorder to confirm it had caught all of that but he managed to keep his hands on the table.

CHAPTER 21

Friday morning, Harrison arrived at International Chest Institute a little after nine. One of the receptionists noticed him enter and made a call.

"How did your deposition go yesterday?" Matt Keys, the leading cardiologist in the small group, asked as he filled the doorway as Hugh was looking at messages on his desk.

"It wasn't fun," he answered. "Long and replete with billable hours."

"Was it nasty?"

"It was just what litigators do."

"How do you feel about it?"

"I think I should sue the attorney who wrote the contracts. He put ambiguous language in a number of locations that I didn't appreciate at the time. Now I'm paying dearly for it."

"We talked about your status here this morning."

"The partners met?"

"We did."

Harrison pointed at a chair and closed the door. His office was small, barely large enough for two, particularly one that weighed almost twice as much as the other. Matt was tall and big, a former collegiate defensive end whose professional prospects snapped along with several knee ligaments. His bright red hair and freckled face blossomed above his giant white coat.

"You've been here over a year. We want you to become a full partner."

"That's nice, flattering in fact."

"We can make the buy-in affordable. Once you have made a commitment and a down payment, your income increases to the partner level."

"How much to buy stock?"

"You would get 5 percent of the company's stock for $350,000. If you pay for it over time out of bonuses, it would take around two years to pay it off." He paused. "Maybe a year and a half, based on your production numbers."

"That's not too different than Chandler."

"I figured it wouldn't be too far off."

"I appreciate you hiring me, Matt. I know we competed pretty hard for years."

"We kept it professional. Your name is good in town, in the whole state, one of the best."

"Thanks."

"And you haven't tried to take over anything, which was a pleasant surprise."

"Only because you could crush me."

They laughed and kidded for a minute, then each went off to work.

Harrison was on call for the weekend. He left the office in the late afternoon after concluding clinic and drove to Samarian Medical Center, where he consulted on a middle-aged woman. Montgomery Pierce, his former partner at Chandler, was seeing a patient in the same department and sat less than twenty feet away, avoiding contact as if Hugh were a leper.

From there, Harrison drove to OCHA for a patient admitted from the emergency department and taken to the CTU, room 4311. At the nursing station, he found Nigel Sampson dictating into the phone, a monotone, rapid, mumbled speech that only God or a transcriptionist could begin to understand. He was among the cohort of doctors whose transcriptions yielded the funniest collections of words.

As Harrison looked through the few chart records, Sampson finished and hung up. "Hi, Hugh. Looks like you pulled the short straw for the weekend, too."

"Once again, into the breech. This cuts into your golf time."

"It would but this weekend looks like rain so I doubt I could get much in. I'll need to go south to get in much playing this late in the season. How's that cute English teacher?"

"She's a lot happier."

"What? Are you engaged?"

"She left."

"Sorry to hear that."

"Sorry to say it. She was refreshing. But, it's over. How is the shoe business?" Sampson's wife had started designing and making shoes several years earlier.

"Erica's making money. She'll need to expand soon."

"Where?"

"She is looking at Arizona. I accepted a job down there near Sedona."

"What?"

"No one knows yet but I'll give the group my resignation on Monday."

"I thought you might be looking at moving somewhere you could golf year round."

"That was one of the decisive points. It's about two hours to Phoenix and less than an hour to Flagstaff. In the summer, golf is great up there, not too hot. Your drives go forty yards farther in that thin air." For a second his eyes looked like golf balls bulging from his pudgy, round face. His white eyelashes made his blue eyes look like a pair of buttons. His fingers twitched as he spoke, a tic Harrison had observed for fifteen years.

"Are you excited about it, Nigel?"

"Chandler ain't what it used to be when we started it up." His right hand rubbed his head as he tilted and twisted his head. He lowered his voice. "Like you, I'm not real comfortable with the tight relationship with this joint."

"It turned out different than I had hoped it would."

"You socialist," he said with a smile. "You sold stock equally to every full partner without retaining a majority for us two to maintaining control."

"I believe that was your position," Harrison retorted with a similar smile.

"Well, you didn't object. I guess maybe we can blame each other for doing the wrong things for all the right reasons."

"Which cliché applies here? The road to hell or the no good deed?"

"Both!" Sampson laughed loud.

A young nurse passed by, shushing him. He watched her sway away and around a corner. Harrison watched his eyes until they turned back to him.

"I'm sorry about this legal mess, Hugh. We should not be talking. After all, you're suing my ass."

"If it were up to you and me, it never would have come to this."

"I know."

"It's amazing how the IQ falls when otherwise intelligent people form a committee."

Sampson laughed again as he stood and stretched. "That was my last patient. I need to get home." He left in his characteristic crab walk, turned slightly right of his path, left arm swinging large and right fingers tapping, arm almost still at his side.

Harrison looked at the ECG and sauntered into room 11. Four hundred and fifty pounds of morbid obesity lay in the bed, his head propped up, struggling to breathe.

Chapter 22

November 2006

"It's been a year and a half and I need the money," yelled Doug Thompson. He, along with Ed and Myra Szabo, met with Dennis Hart.

"I understand, Douglas. I do." Hart kept his professional demeanor. "This is a painfully slow process, as I told you at the start. We are now at the point where we can turn the screws."

"You've dropped so many people from the complaint," Myra complained. "Won't that mean less money?"

"The intensivist and the internists did nothing wrong by any standard. Keeping them in weakens our case." His conference room could have been any in hundreds of cities: walls lined with case law books, cherry wood veneer table, round-backed cushioned chairs, glass doors, plush carpets and a view of the city. "Their cardiology expert is weak. They had to find one that would say both the cardiologists were right when they used opposite approaches. Our experts are top guns from big academic centers, Stanford, Johns Hopkins, and the Cleveland Clinic. Their statements are strong and on deposition they were stunning. We will win if we go to trial. They will settle before then."

"How long will that take?" Doug asked.

"A couple of months, I think."

"I need the money now," he said.

"The only way you will get any money sooner is to settle for a small fraction of what I see coming. Did you read the forensic accountant's report?"

"Hell no."

"You should look at it, Doug," Ed interjected.

"Why don't you just give me the *Reader's Digest* version?"

"Sarah died at age thirty-four," Hart began. "If she retired at age sixty-six, the current expectation, she was deprived of thirty-two years of income. Her income averaged one hundred eighty thousand a year from 1997 to 1999. Multiply that by thirty-two and you get five and a half million dollars as the minimum loss. Add attorney fees, court costs and correct for anticipated inflation and it's close to ten million. That does not include a punitive award, typically treble damages. We are asking thirty million, based on the accountant's numbers."

"And I thought you just pulled that number out of your ass."

"Doug!" Myra scolded.

"If you settle immediately," Hart removed his reading glasses, "you might get ten to fifty thousand dollars."

"We are not going to settle for that," Myra asserted, pointing her nose slightly upward.

"I won't have no cash until the resorts open. It don't look too good right now."

"It will take months to work out a settlement, Douglas. We can't simply say send us a check for X dollars. That's not how it works." Hart strained to be patient.

"I'm getting evicted unless I make some rent payments."

"Amy will be fine with us," Ed said. "We're already taking her most days."

"Ed!" Myra exclaimed. "We have a small, fixed income. I can't even afford my pills."

"You have the life insurance and I need money now!" Doug raised his voice.

Ed rolled his eyes. They still had close to a million dollars from Sarah's life insurance in an account for Amy. He had arranged access only for himself and wouldn't allow Myra to even see the balance. Doug and Myra started talking over each other resulting in brief mayhem.

"STOP!" Mr. Hart tried to regain some degree of order. "You have made the point that time is of the essence. I will put more pressure on the defendants and the liability company. It is clear we need to bring this to a successful conclusion in a hurry."

"Amen to that," Doug agreed.

A few minutes later, in his office Hart dictated a note and a letter with his eyes on the nine million-dollar contingency fee for his firm.

Chapter 23

Monday, November 25, Brady Hicks woke up at 5:30 and started to get ready for work as a security guard at the Salt Lake City International Airport. He was sipping coffee from a travel mug in his old Nissan truck when he noticed a burning deep in his chest. The coffee had cooled a little since he left home. He took a few more swallows and the discomfort increased. Driving with his left hand he fumbled with his lunch sack and pulled out a cookie. It made no improvement. The discomfort became a pain. Prickly heat erupted on his brow bringing beads of sweat. Water ran down his chest underneath his uniform. His neck ached. So did both upper arms, especially his left. His truck swerved as he became lightheaded. He took the first exit he could find, which was a mile or so away from OCHA. It was not the hospital covered by his managed care. That realization caused only momentary hesitation but increased his anxiety.

Wiping perspiration from his eyes he tromped on the accelerator. Driving with one hand he loosened the buttons on his shirt, now dark and wet. He growled with pain, gritting his teeth, forcing his mind to focus on driving. He pulled into the emergency drive, feeling like his chest was ready to explode. Blackness edged in from the sides and top of his vision. His foot flapped for the brake as a tunnel of light became smaller until it was a pinpoint. Then gone.

The truck swerved, slowing down as the driver slumped behind the wheel, held upright only by the shoulder harness. It stopped when it plowed into an ambulance. Two uniformed personnel had unloaded a stretcher carrying a bundled, white-haired patient. They were barely bumped in the collision but startled by the noise. The female attendant cursed. The medic looked inside the Nissan and popped the door open. The driver did not react; his eyes open in a dead stare. The medic released Hick's seatbelt and pulled him to the pavement.

"We have a code here!" he bellowed and felt in vain for a pulse. His partner left the old patient alone and called into the hospital emergency room. She came to help and was followed by three personnel from inside. A defibrillator showed Hicks was in a cardiac arrest. One shock was delivered. He twitched painfully, arching and falling in a fraction of a second after fifty thousand volts coursed through his body. His rhythm normalized and within ten seconds he had a palpable pulse. The ECG showed injury but a good rhythm. He also had a pulse. He took a sonorous breath followed slowly by another. They lifted him onto a stretcher and hurried him inside, placing him in the cardiac room, still unconscious.

Wallace Walton, tired and looking forward to ending his overnight shift, was the emergency room physician. He assessed Hicks as they took blood pressure, did an ECG and extracted his wallet to find his name and age, fifty-two.

"Who's on call for cardiology?" he asked into the intercom.

"Harrison."

"Call him, STAT."

Hicks began to stir and wake up, flailing with his arms, kicking with his legs, twisting his head away from the face mask giving him oxygen.

"Should we sedate him, Doctor?" one of the three nurses taking care of him asked.

"He'll stop once he wakes up. Give it a few minutes."

"Dr. Harrison on line twenty-two." This came out of the speaker on the wall.

"Walton. Hi, Hugh. Do you have your cathing shoes on?"

"What's up?" Harrison looked at the clock on the wall of his kitchen. In theory he was not on call for another ten minutes.

"We have a fifty-two-year-old guy who had a cardiac arrest in our driveway and mangled an ambulance with the truck he was driving. We shocked him once for V fib. His ECG now shows an acute anterior MI. He is waking up and has reasonable vital signs. BP is 110."

"Do you any other history?"

"No. He hasn't said anything, just groans."

"Let's call the cath lab. I'll be there in fifteen minutes."

"Do you want us to give him anything?"

"Aspirin, if he can swallow, and heparin IV."

The call ended. The clerk called the hospital operator to page the cardiac catheterization laboratory crew.

The regular day shift people were arriving. Two nurses had been dispatched to bring down an elective patient of Malouf as two others prepared the room, opening sterile equipment needed and placing it on the sterile table.

Harrison arrived about ten minutes after seven and went directly to examine Hicks. He was awake but under the influence of morphine, speech slurred, lids heavy and still in a lot of pain. Hugh asked a dozen questions, listened to his heart and lungs and came to the nursing station. Wally stood there wearing a golf cap and windbreaker.

"I'm out of here," Wally said. "Anything you need from me?"

"Is the cath lab coming?"

Wally pointed at the clerk, who also started work ten minutes earlier. He nodded and said, "I'll call."

Wally left and Hugh listened to the clerk call as he scribbled a brief note. "'ello. Dees ees Jorge in the emergency room." Harrison hoped that whoever was on the other end of the call could understand the thick accent. "Are you aware dah we have an acute MI down here who need a STAT cat? No, an acute MI. Yes, he need cat now. Dr. Harrison. No. Yes. Yes. Just a minute. Doctor, they want to speak with you."

He took the phone, lifting the base to the counter where he was writing and stretching the kinked cord. "Harrison here."

"We just heard about the acute. We are getting a patient of Malouf's on the table right now. Do we need to take this lady back to her room?"

"Yes. This is a big anterior who's had one cardiac arrest already."

"Can you call Dr. Malouf?"

"I'm on the move. I'll call her when I get to the lab."

"Malouf will scream if we take her patient off the table."

"Get her off. Malouf knows the rules. I'll be right there."

He hung up and hurried in. The ECG tracing on the monitor showed the chaotic line of a cardiac arrest. Hicks looked dead. The nurse was operating the defibrillator.

"Clear!" she called as she charged the machine.

A warning whine increased in pitch. No one touched the bed as the nurse waved her hand like a roulette attendant stopping the betting. She pushed the lighted red button. Hicks arched and fell, arms flying up. A few seconds later the ECG line drifted out of the top of the screen where it had disappeared and resumed a normal rhythm. He moaned and clutched his chest.

"Get him ready to roll to the lab. I'm headed over there now. Give him 150 milligrams of amiodarone IV." He wanted to prevent additional cardiac arrests with the drug.

Harrison hurried to the cath lab. A woman who appeared to be about forty-five or fifty was on a stretcher, nervous and distressed in the hall outside the room. He went inside the control room.

"Would you page Malouf for me?"

A technician was entering information into one of several computers for the emergency case. "I'm on it," he said as he tapped a button on the phone, waited for a signal and entered the pager number and a send key. "I'll be changing," he said as he left and went to the locker room. It was a room with a bench in the middle and a large number of metal lockers. His had a shamrock. He spun the combination dial and jerked the handle up twice before it opened. He was standing in his white striped boxer shorts when the intercom screeched. "Dr. Malouf on line two."

"Sarisha, this is Hugh. I have a fifty-two-year-old with an MI in the ER. I need to bump your first case."

"I'm across the hall. Be there in a minute."

Click.

As he tied a double knot in the string that held his scrub pants up he heard a commotion in the hall. He slipped into his clogs and a scrub top, grabbed his wallet, phone and pager and exited.

"How many times have I told you morons not ever, ever, EVER to take my patient off the table without my express permission?" Malouf was yelling at the staff with the patient a few feet away and enrapt in the confrontation.

"I told them to do it," Harrison said.

"If this is not a bona fide emergency, I'll have your privileges pulled."

"Ooo. The mighty and powerful Malouf." Harrison feigned fear momentarily. "My patient has arrested twice and has a huge anterior MI by ECG. So, cool down." He went to walk past but Malouf put her hand on his chest and halted him.

"Nobody takes my patient off the table. Nobody."

Harrison rolled his eyes and sighed. "Don't denigrate me."

"I'll bet your patient would gladly help to save his life by delaying the procedure," he said loudly enough for the elderly patient to hear. "Besides, you know the rules."

"You're an ass!"

He tried to move past but, as he did so, Malouf shoved hard with both hands. Off balance, he stumbled a few steps, then fell, breaking his fall with his left hand. The patient, watching this, audibly inhaled in surprise and fear. Two nurses rushed over to where Hugh fell. He was already getting up, grimacing. The little finger on his left hand took an unexpected turn and was angled away from the others.

The patient screamed. The nurses gasped. Malouf gaped in guilt.

Harrison looked at the finger from a couple of angles. Then, he grasped it and pulled it straight.

The patient screamed again.

"Dr. Harrison!" one of the nurses yelled. "What are you doing?"

"I have a case to do."

"It could be broken. You need an X-ray."

This time when he went to pass Malouf she backed away. He said nothing. He heard the rhythmic beeping of a heart monitor grow louder. He poked his head inside the room. "Our patient is here," he said.

Nurses whisked Hicks into the lab.

Malouf's elderly patient sat up and twisted her feet off the stretcher. "I want a different doctor!"

She pulled her gown around so her bare backside was covered, hopped off and started walking. One of the nurses left in pursuit. Malouf went as well.

Harrison's little finger was maroon and growing. He tried to flex. He winced. "I don't think I can do this case," he said to Debbie, a nurse.

She stayed right by him as he went back to the control booth.

"Can you page Keys?" He sat down, keeping his finger up.

"I'll get some ice," Debbie said.

"What happened?" asked Brent, the technician.

"Dislocated my finger."

The ice came in and he soon held a plastic bag in a washcloth against his injury. The finger was bigger than the adjacent ring finger and throbbing. Keys had not called back.

The clock was running and time was muscle. The faster the blocked artery got opened, the better the patient would do. Hugh couldn't wait. He put on his lead apron, hat and mask and walked to the sink and carefully washed his hands.

Less than ten minutes later, he had found not only a blocked anterior artery but severe narrowing of the left main, the "widow maker" artery, a dilemma he faced rarely. The left main was so narrow that the balloon he had to push into the left anterior descending would plug it off.

"Should we call surgery?" Debbie asked.

"No."

"Are you sure?"

"It'll take way too long. He has a better chance if I just fix both now."

Surgery was typically done for left main artery narrowing but this applied to elective surgery, not in a sick, acute heart attack patient. Half an hour later, Hugh took off his gloves, unable to feel his left little finger anymore because the combination of swelling and the constriction of the glove. He filled out orders, wrote a note then went to talk to the family. Hicks was groggy from narcotics and perhaps from a few periods of very low blood pressure during the procedure. Afterward he returned to a small room near the lab to dictate the history and physical and the procedure note.

Debbie and Brent wheeled Hicks from the lab to the elevator, picking up his wife and a few family members on the way.

"Doctor says you're going to be okay, Brady," his wife, Andrea, gushed as she kissed his cool, damp forehead.

He said nothing, just tried to smile.

"How did it go in there?" a woman holding Andrea's arm asked Debbie.

"Didn't Dr. Harrison talk to you?" she replied as the elevator door opened.

"He did," she said. "He said it went well but I thought he was being kind instead of telling what actually happened."

"Who are you?" Debbie asked.

"I'm sorry," Andrea said. "This is my sister, Mel."

"We had to resuscitate him a couple of times. It was a little dicey," Brent said.

"You are really lucky that you got Dr. Harrison," Debbie said. "I don't think that many others would have got him through this so well. He's amazing with sick patients."

"You mean, he almost died in there?" Andrea asked.

Mel hugged her.

"He had a problem that we usually send for surgery because they are so dangerous," Debbie said. "We call them *widow-makers*. It's a good thing he fixed it because it closed completely before we got a wire in it. He might have died going for surgery."

"Thank you so much."

"Thank Dr. Harrison," Brent said. "He broke his finger just before we started and still ... One more thing to add to the legend."

The elevator door opened and they wheeled the bed into the cardiac ICU. Mel pulled out a little notebook and wrote down everything she remembered from the short conversation.

His dictations done, Harrison hesitated for several minutes then punched nine for the outside line, then nine, one, one.

"I would like to report an assault." He explained the situation to the operator, who said an officer would meet him in the emergency room.

By that time, Debbie was back and checked on Harrison's swollen finger. She called the lab manager, who said she would call the cardiology service line director, who probably would push the report of the fight to up the chain of command up to Don Zone, chief executive officer. Debbie walked him to the ER.

While Harrison was getting his hand X-rayed, two policemen interviewed Debbie and Alisha, who witnessed the altercation. They spoke to the ER doc, then to Harrison. Debbie and Alecia guided them to the cath lab, where Sarisha was arrested for assault when she emerged from the cath lab. A videographer for a local TV station recorded Dr. Malouf in handcuffs, leaving the front door of OCHA and being assisted into a police car. As the news spread rapidly throughout the hospital, there were high-fives, low-fives and knuckle kisses. It could not have happened to a bigger bitch, they agreed.

As expected there was a small corner of bone knocked off at the dislocation, technically the *left fifth proximal interphalangeal joint*. Surgery would not be needed but his finger would be splinted for weeks. This would keep him away from doing any procedures.

In the late afternoon while Harrison was at the Chest Institute office reading echocardiograms and nuclear stress tests done earlier in the day, he received a phone call.

"Dr. Harrison, this is Monica Jessop. Do you have a minute?"

"For you, yes."

"We just received a hand-delivered envelope from Dennis Hart. Are you sitting down?"

"Oh, the drama."

"I'm not kidding."

"Go ahead." Hugh backed away from the computer screen and turned up the lights. He turned over a blank form so he could take notes.

"We have an amended complaint. They dropped everyone but you, Dr. Blackstone, Chandler Cardiovascular and Olympus. They are asking thirty million dollars."

"Whoa. Thirty million? Where did that come from?"

"Lost income projection, attorney fees and punitive damages."

"That goes way beyond my malpractice coverage limit."

"I know that."

"They could take everything I own and garnish my wages, assuming I could even practice after that."

"Don't get upset. You'd have to lose first."

"Hard not to let that bother me."

"Also, just to let you know, they want an expedited trial because Amy Thompson, the little girl with Down syndrome, needs therapy that her mother would have provided were she alive with her previous income potential."

"Did she not have life insurance?"

"Yes, but not even close to what they want. And it's irrelevant for this case."

"Well, Monica, this is awful."

"Unfortunately, for a jury trial they have a huge advantage, the premature death of a young and successful professional whose orphaned child has lifelong special needs. WIE thinks we should propose a mediation to settle this."

"We thinks?"

"Sorry, WIE, Western Insurance Exchange, your liability insurance company and the attorneys that represent Blackstone and the hospital."

"She had giant cell myocarditis. It's one hundred percent fatal. I have to pay for that?"

"They claim she would be alive today but for your errors."

"What? That I failed to send a stable patient to a hospital with worse outcomes in heart failure?" He stood at his desk, almost yelling into the phone. "It was Blackstone who made her crash, then held on to her until she was unsalvageable."

"And you can't say that. You and he have the same malpractice carrier."

"I can't defend myself?"

"That's *my* job, Dr. Harrison."

"Sounds like you're working for the insurance company. They're paying you." Sam was trying not to sound angry. It wasn't working out too well.

"They pay me to defend you."

"I should pay my own lawyer."

"That'd be a mistake. WIE won't have to cover your losses if you do."

"What?"

"Fine print. You should read it sometime."

Harrison exhaled in frustration but said nothing. There was an awkward silence until Jessop spoke.

"I'll keep you informed about where this is headed. You should receive a copy of the latest amended complaint in the mail."

When she ended the call, Harrison slid the handset into the cradle and stared at a wall as blank as his thoughts.

CHAPTER 24

International Chest Institute was empty except for a small cleaning crew and Hugh Harrison. He called attorney Anthony Joseph Dominici, an attorney of Higgins Cowen, the largest whistleblower, or *qui tam*, law firm in the United States. After hearing he could lose $10 million, fear eased his hesitation about contacting this firm. After the pleasantries, the discussion turned to business at hand.

Harrison explained the details as he knew them of the agreement between his former practice and OCHA.

"We'll need to review that contract," Dominici said.

"I got it in discovery for the lawsuit between them and me with the stipulation it could be used only for that purpose."

"I still need to see it. Fax it and maybe we can find a way around their gag order."

"Okay."

"I've heard this song before, same chorus, different verse." Dominici's voice was tenor and smooth. Hugh had never met the man. "Suspicious Healthcare, as we call them around here, has had similar agreements before that were found to be illegal. They've had multiple fines for millions of dollars and forced to enter into a consent decree with the Justice department wherein they committed to avoid similar arrangements with physicians in the future. Our firm brought the last infraction to the attention of the authorities that resulted in the fine."

"How much money did your firm make?"

"We won that one but the nature of *qui tam* is risky. These are highly technical matters and require a great deal of work. We take only those cases where we think the potential reward is worth the risk of spending a lot on assets on a losing cause."

"What do you think about this situation?"

"On the one hand, the amount of money the government has lost due to this agreement is not huge, so Justice may not be excessively upset. However, this would be the first violation since the consent decree with Auspicious. If I were a government attorney, I would hit them with an enormous fine, despite the fairly small amount of loss due to the breech. I would like very much to continue to investigate this."

"You have no idea how happy that makes me." Harrison immediately regretted the uncharacteristic optimism but it just flashed out from the little glimmer of financial hope.

"I said *investigate*. We have not decided to pursue the matter. The next steps are to review all the documents we can, review recent awards, do some estimate as to whether this is financially worthwhile for us and, if all that looks favorable, meet with your local US attorney. Think it over tonight and if you're still willing to proceed, send me an email to that effect tomorrow. I'll then make plans to fly out with one or two of my associates. Remember, Dr. Harrison, that when the trouble hits, it will hit hard. OCHA may do everything it can to get you off staff. Your friends and colleagues may turn against you. You will be criticized and slandered. There may be threats. It can get very ugly, so much so that many whistleblowers give up. We need some assurance from you that you are willing to persevere, which is why I want to give you a little time to consider."

"These people have done harm to me personally and to the community in general. I'm not backing down."

"Good. It will be nice to meet face to face."

"Is there any benefit in naming Chandler Cardiovascular Clinic?"

"They don't have the deep pockets. It increases our expenses without much chance to recoup. Obviously they are not part of the consent decree but they have colluded in perpetrating fraud against the United States of America and have benefitted enormously by so doing, it would appear. We'll need to think about it."

"I would like to include them. If nothing else, it would serve notice to all such groups not to collude and cheat."

"It's a noble thought. We'll consider it," Dominici said.

The call ended. He tidied his desk and headed home earlier than usual. Thanksgiving week was usually slower than normal. It was trying to snow, tiny flakes giving texture to a stiff cold breeze.

Dominici had probably figured out the reason for including his former group was a vendetta. The throbbing in his finger was a constant reminder of the fight between him and his old partners. Between the Lortab now in his stomach, the leverage he now had over Sarisha Malouf, and the possibility of a huge fine against Chandler, his pains were beginning to ease.

Chapter 25

Earlier that afternoon Ed Szabo parked across the street from Winkler in a church parking lot. He found Amy waiting at the front door, received her usual enthusiastic greeting and took the longer walk back to the car for a little extra exercise. He drove to Doug's apartment. A while after he knocked Doug came to the door in a ragged wife-beater undershirt, hitching up his pants. A Native American woman in a bathrobe leaned against the doorframe in the darkness smoking a joint. Ed and Amy entered. Doug went into the hall and came out with a box of Amy's things and put it on the floor. He returned to the back and brought out a black plastic garbage bag full of clothing.

"That's it," Doug said. "Those are Amy's things."

The woman shifted as she blew smoke at the ceiling. Her robe fell partially open and she smiled at Ed with gold-edged teeth.

"Yah-ta-hey," Ed said in an effort to be culturally sensitive.

"Hey, Ruby's Blackfeet, not Navaho, Ed."

"Sorry."

Ed lifted the box and bounced off the frame to exit the house. Doug carried the bag and Amy followed Doug. They put Amy's possessions in the trunk of the Camry.

Doug gave her a brief hug. "You're gonna stay with Grandma and Grandpa for a while until I get more money."

"I like it there," she said and coughed.

"Bye-bye, babe," Doug said.

She picked her nose and got in the car. Ed drove away, muttering angrily about the toxic environment for his granddaughter.

"What's spitty?" she asked.

"I'm sorry. Just talking to myself." It was a reminder to watch his language.

The next morning, Tuesday, the wind had died and cold settled in. A few inches of snow had fallen making the roads slick. Ed arrived about 6:00, an hour earlier than usual. He took a break to drive Amy to school and went inside with her. He asked the principle a few questions about marijuana and kids. She called Child Protective Services and together they asked a few questions.

The officer gave Ed the address for the crime lab and an appointment that afternoon to collect some hair from Amy to assess for exposure before doing anything else.

After school Ed took Amy for a ride to the lab on the west side of the valley.

All Tuesday morning through clinic, Harrison was trying to figure out how he could do a cardiac catheterization with a splint on his finger. His contracts attorney, Leo Damjanovich, called in the late morning and arranged to meet midafternoon, the time made possible by his injury. There was a decision from the judge about the breach of contract that needed some discussion. Plus Gullimore had called him about an assault. Damjanovich needed details.

Dingle and Damjanovich was not a large firm but occupied one entire floor in the Boston Building. Harrison arrived a few minutes late.

"What happened to your finger?" Damjanovich asked, noticing the bright white bandage.

"Malouf shoved me. I fell and dislocated one of the joints."

"All ninety pounds of her?" He grinned. "Must be tough."

"I wasn't expecting her to attack."

They walked to a small conference room, picking up a cup of tea on the way. Leo left the door ajar.

"The judge dismissed the largest of your three claims, almost half of what we're asking, the stock issue. I believe his decision goes against precedent but that is what he decided."

"I thought that was pretty weak anyway, so I can't say I'm too surprised."

"I'm weighing the pros and cons of an appeal but for the moment this takes a lot of wind out of our sails, Dr. Harrison." Leo pushed his glasses higher on his long and angular nose and squirmed for relief from his light blue shirt collar. "It's a momentum changer."

"The other claims are intact?"

"Yes, but he recommended that we take the case to an arbitrator."

"Instead of wasting his time?"

"So it seems."

"Arbitrator? What does that mean?"

"They are typically expert attorneys that look at the facts and the position of both sides and make a judgement. It can be binding, meaning the decision is final. They tend to split the pain, unlike a court where it's usually one side wins all. The arbitrator could take the loss of stock into consideration even though the judge has thrown it out."

"Sounds like you're in favor."

"I think the judge will not like it if we block his great idea. On the other hand, I got a call from Gullimore fishing for a deal. Now that I know about your run in with Malouf, it makes some sense."

"So it had something to do with the misdemeanor assault charge against Malouf."

"He didn't mention any criminal charges. Have you filed?"

"Not yet."

"Good. He said if the personal matter between you two could be amicably put away they would be willing to settle fairly on the remaining claims. Can you give me more detail about what happened and what charges have been made?"

Harrison outlined the events.

"Will your injury impair your ability to do your job?"

"For now. Not sure about permanent function but I doubt it'll make any difference."

"Have you seen a hand surgeon?"

"Not yet. Next week."

"Are you working?"

"I had clinic all morning."

"If you work, you're not disabled."

"If a surgeon can't operate, is he disabled? I can only clinical work, no procedures probably for about a month. The bulk of my income is procedures."

"Would you be willing to drop charges against her if we get a good settlement?"

"The county attorney might choose not to pursue this if the police investigation doesn't support it, so they said."

"That'd be a shame."

"And a month or so of reduced income doesn't support a large settlement."

"I'll work up something this afternoon and see if we can't get the whole matter resolved before committing to arbitration."

Harrison's pager sounded. He checked the message. "I should probably get back to the hospital."

Chapter 26

Ed slipped out of work early chased by a raft of "banker's hours" epithets. He picked up Amy and drove to the crime lab. A young woman was wearing dark bell-bottom slacks and an off-white swiped her ID over the charcoal-colored security reader next to the door and brought them inside. The technologist snipped a few long hairs from Amy's head.

"That's all the hair I need," she said.

"One more thing," Ed said. "Her dad had her tattooed on her bottom."

"Fluff-fly!" Amy said with a smile.

"I don't think that's against the law," she said. "But I could take a picture of it if you'd like. I also need fingerprints for a more complete ID."

Amy exposed the butterfly and the woman took several photographs. They walked into an adjacent room and obtained fingerprints on a scanner. A printer produced a copy on which Amy scribbled her initials.

On the way home, the sun was lower and the traffic thicker.

"Amy," Ed said. "Do you know what a secret is?"

"Yes."

"What is it?"

"Something you don't tell."

"Right. What we did after school is a secret. Neither of us can tell Grandma or your dad or anyone. Is that okay?"

"We have secret." A conspiratorial look fell over her face. "Okay, Gwamps."

"Pinky swear?" He held out his little finger.

She giggled and extended her own, wrapping it around.

"Pinky swear," she said as they bounced up and down three times, making this a most solemn oath.

The rest of the way home he tried to get her to say "Grandpa" correctly.

When they arrived, Myra was not in her chair in front of the television, a bit unusual.

"Myra?" Ed called a couple of times before he heard something from the bathroom.

The fecal and uriniferous odors met him before he found her lying still on the floor.

"Good God!" She gasped, turning her eyes and head just enough to see him. "Where have you been? I can't get up."

He tried to hold her hands and help her up but she fell. "I'm worn out, you idiot."

He stepped behind her, into the tub, crouched and put his arms under hers and locked his hands under her wet breasts. It was only sweat, he hoped. He lifted and inched her up against the side of the tub until she could get her legs underneath. The stench made him retch. Pulling with all his might he couldn't get her up to the edge of tub. He stopped, both of them panting heavily. On the floor was a puddle of urine. Ed steadied her until he thought she would not tip over. He carefully stepped out and hit the fan switch then the spray can of deodorizer.

"Damn it, Ed. What took you so long?"

"How much do you weigh, Myra?"

"I have no idea."

"I'm going to call the paramedics."

"No, you're not."

He left the bathroom and made the call.

He found a wooden milking stool, sturdy and small in the garage. He put it next to her but still could not get her off the floor. The effort and smells were too much. Ed lost his lunch into the toilet bowl.

"Great," Myra said. "You're quite the man."

Ed rinsed out his mouth and went to the front door. No emergency vehicles yet, he saw. Back inside, Amy sat on the floor, her legs splayed, watching cartoons. Her belly protruded from under her tight shirt and her developing breasts were augmented by her excess weight. He vowed to put her on a diet and get her more exercise. For the moment, she was fine.

Back in the bathroom, Myra had tipped over onto the three-legged stool, her consciousness flagging. He eased her down to the floor and by that time there were loud knocks on the door.

He let two firemen in and saw a paramedic rig pull up. Twenty minutes later, she was on a gurney and into an ambulance, griping whenever she was conscious that this was all a big bother.

He returned to clean the bathroom, thinking if they got only one tenth of what they were asking in this lawsuit, he would take his share and leave. He thought of living in Mesquite or Reno, Nevada, or in a motor home for as long as he had gas money. The room, their marriage, his job all stunk. But then there is Amy. She was the one bright spot in his life. She needed him and he needed her. He scrubbed until he had made the room sparkle and smell like hypochlorite.

After he finished, he bundled up Amy and they drove to the hospital. In the emergency department Myra was awake and cleaned up, two IV lines running clear fluid into her veins.

"I have to be here overnight," was her grumpy greeting.

"Okay."

"They have to run tests. If you'd been home, this wouldn't have happened."

"You would've fallen anyway."

"I wouldn't have been stuck there for hours. It makes me so angry. Why don't you retire?"

She wouldn't like the real answer. Instead of saying that spending more time with her would be intolerable, he said nothing. Amy hugged his arm, seeming fearful.

Myra threw her hands in the air and grunted. "Come, Amy," she said, patting a sliver of bed next to her.

Amy didn't budge.

A nurse came in, puttered around with the ECG monitor and the IV pumps, looked over the patient and left.

"Amy needs dinner and to get to bed," Ed said. "We're going to leave."

"That was awfully short," she fumed.

After picking up some fast food they got home. Ed put Amy to bed then escaped to the tiny patio with a Pabst Blue Ribbon. It would stay cool in the night chill.

The next day Ed got a call from the Child Protective Services officer he spoke with the day before.

"Amy's father, Doug Thompson, was pulled over for erratic driving and arrested. His blood alcohol level was 0.14, well over the limit."

"When?"

"About midnight. This was his fourth arrest for the same problem, so his license is suspended. I thought you ought to know for Amy's sake."

"Like I said, she's been exposed to second-hand marijuana smoke and God knows what else. Doug is a troubled guy."

"Police also found a small bag of marijuana in the purse of a woman, Ruby Blackfeather of Heart Butte, Montana, who was with him at the time. Doug, of course, claimed that he knew nothing about it despite smoke inside the car."

"I'm just glad he had the good sense of letting her stay here."

"Does she stay with you often?"

"Most of the time, to be honest."

"Are you okay with assuming full guardianship?"

"Of course. He's been a terrible father."

"Thanks. That's good to know when we review this situation. He's in jail, now. Are you able to care for her for the time being?"

"I'd like to get him out of her life, at least as far as parenting is concerned and take over all of it myself, er, ourselves."

CHAPTER 27

Shortly after 5:00 and the office was rapidly emptying. Harrison chatted with an echo tech on the way out when Matt Keys called out from his office. Hugh came in.

"Nice finger," Keys said. "Makes it hard to do pelvic exams."

"Thank God I don't," Harrison answered.

"I don't look at vaginas that way, either." He smiled.

"So, are we here to discuss the pros and cons of the female perineum?"

"I want to hear what you think about our offer."

"I talked to my accountant. He asked me, 'How much do you want to join this group?' He pointed out that I and the other shareholders would be required to buy back stock of those that leave. When you leave it would cost me and the three others about a quarter of a million bucks each. So, not only do I pay something like three hundred fifty K for my shares now, I'm on the hook to buy back stock from everyone that leaves before I do. It's not worth it."

"It would be the same for you when you sell your stock, Hugh."

"I see that. I would rather stay on as an employed physician."

"That's not an option."

"What?"

Keys leaned back and placed both hands behind his head, displaying sweat marks in the armpits of his gray shirt. "We need everyone in the practice to be fully invested. You're a good cardiologist, better than everyone else here but me." He smiled at his own hubris. "If you won't buy in, we'll terminate your employment when the current contract ends December 31."

"I thought it was going to be extended."

"I changed my mind. And we increased the price to $400,000."

"I signed the agreement."

"I didn't." He leaned forward. "I'd like you to stay, Hugh. I really would. You have a great work ethic. You care about covering the service and keeping the practice growing. You'll benefit from being an owner. You should reconsider."

"I'm not going to fund your retirement. That's what your buy-sell agreement does."

"I have $3 million or so in my retirement plan already," Keys said with a smile.

"Ten times more than I've got, thanks to divorce."

"Buy in and you'll be fine."

"It's not fine that you give me, in essence, five weeks' notice that I won't have a job, Matt. I signed that extension months ago."

"Buy in, then. Just say yes. That's what you always tell us."

"I don't bend to coercion. Have a nice life. I have three weeks of vacation built up. You won't see me after about December 10."

"You won't be able to fund your war against Chandler, Hugh."

Harrison walked out.

"You're on call over Christmas, Hugh."

"No, I'm on vacation unless you pay me $5,000 a day for call."

Harrison stormed out of the office and took a circuitous route home. No amount of thinking was going to change the offer and the financial consequences.

Beth Savery's car was in his driveway. She was an endodontist and they had been dating for a few months. When Hugh entered his home, the smell of basil filled the air and clanking came from the kitchen. Strainers, pans, bowls, spatulas and spoons were piled in the sink. In a tight red sweater, sleeves pulled up to her elbows, Beth grated cheese.

"Dr. Savery! What are you doing?"

"Slaving over your food," she grinned, turning to give a profile of her augmented chest. "I hope you haven't eaten."

"No."

"This is a South Beach Diet night."

"What's that?"

"A low carbohydrate plan for weight loss, developed by a cardiologist just like you except much richer, I would guess."

"That would depend on how many ex-wives he has."

"Funny."

"Are you telling me I'm fat?"

"We could both stand to lose a few pounds, you know."

She whirred into a kitchen frenzy as Hugh hustled into his office and dropped his briefcase and a handful of mail.

When he returned, four tall candles burned and his heated plate held pink salmon, fried long green beans and a baked half tomato covered with pesto. "This looks fabulous," he said in awe. "Amazing."

Her hair that had been held in a scrunchy when he entered was now brushed and luxurious. "How was your day?"

"I've had better. First, I met with Leo. The big-money part of my lawsuit was thrown out by the judge. That was most of my case." He savored the salmon, finishing the first bite with a sip of chilled chardonnay.

"Sorry to hear that. How's is your finger?"

"It's sore. How was your day of root canals?"

"Only three. Mostly it was pre and post visits. We blew through a huge schedule, didn't even have time to talk on the phone."

"You must be tired."

"It's a lot of work."

"I got fired today," he stated as he raised his glass. "To life!"

Beth blinked in confusion. "Hugh! You what?"

"If I don't accept the offer to be a shareholder of ICI, my employment will end on New Year's Eve."

"Is that your decision?"

"Theirs."

"I thought you had signed an extension. Can they do that?"

"Probably. Matt said he did not sign my new contract. I was wondering why I hadn't seen it since I signed. He might have waited to create more pressure for me to become an owner. To life!" He gestured with his glass again.

"I'm not drinking to that," Beth said. "This is horrible news and you're hiding the pain beneath a facade of celebration."

"You're right."

"What are you going to do?"

"I don't know." Hugh spoke as he swirled his glass, studying the wine legs and the deep red meniscus. "Options are to try to join another group in town, probably impossible at this point, or to start a solo practice and build it up like I did with Chandler. I could try to find a job in another town or out of state. That would take quite a while plus it takes months to get another medical license."

"I bet a lot of your patients would follow you."

Beth stirred around in her food as Hugh each bite with a swallow from his goblet, refilling it frequently.

"I'll need to open another bottle," Beth remarked.

"Not for me. I'm switching to Scotch after this glass."

"I don't like how your breath smells when you've had whiskey."

"C'est la vie."

Beth tightened up. "I don't think you're going to be good company tonight," she said.

Not long after dinner, Beth went home.

A letter signed by Matt Keys, M.D., lay orthogonally positioned on Hugh's desk when he arrived at his office at seven o'clock Wednesday morning. It stated simply that his contract would not be renewed, that effective January first he would not be employed. Harrison dropped it in his International Chest Institute file and walked to OCHA.

CHAPTER 28

Doctors Blackstone and Pierce met with Malouf in her office early Wednesday.

"We won part of the summary judgment," Malouf boasted. "Harrison's claim is cut in half. I told Gullimore to see if he could settle."

"First, Sarisha, tell me about the fight you two had," Pierce said, glowering.

"It was not a fight." She had practiced the explanation and memorized a speech about it. She controlled her posture and gestures to exude calm and confidence with no hint of guilt or apology. She laughed and waved her hand dismissively. "We were having a verbal disagreement. He tripped and fell and ended up on the ground with his little finger sticking out at a right angle. He must have called the cops later and accused me of assault. Ridiculous."

"Were you booked?"

"It was demeaning."

"Your version is not the one that is circulating around the hospital," Blackstone said.

"I honestly think he took a fall on purpose to make it appear that I hit him."

"He filed charges?"

"Pending, as I understand."

"Do you have a criminal defense attorney?" Pierce asked.

"Of course I do, Monty."

Pierce stroked his jowls as he drilled with his pale blue eyes. "When will you be arraigned?"

"I believe the charges will be dropped."

"Oh?" Pierce leaned closer. "Why would you think that? Are you and Hugh tight?"

"I told Gullimore to explore what it would take to get him to drop the charges."

"Are you crazy?" Blackstone spurted. "You want us to pay for your sin?" She saw he tried and failed to keep religion out of it.

"You had no authorization to say that, Sarisha," Pierce objected.

"I didn't think I needed any."

"It's our money, not yours," he continued. "If we paid, say, $100,000 extra to get you off the hook, that means almost $10,000 out of the pocket of every doc in the practice."

"We've paid a lot of money over the years to smooth over problems created by several of us, haven't we, Stan?" Malouf smiled, the gap between her front teeth giving her the look of an evil cat again. He looked away in embarrassment.

"Our attorney gutted Harrison's claim then you screw up and give him more leverage."

Pierce's voice was loud. Blackstone leaned back and latched the door.

"We could win this outright and you offer to settle? Without asking permission from the board? Come on, Sarisha, what are you thinking?"

After letting that sink in, Pierce continued. "You should call Gullimore back and tell him no quarter. Go for the jugular. No camel trading, no negotiations, no compromises. Harrison broke his agreement. We paid him what the contract demanded and we want our legal fees back. Period."

"Camel trading? Seriously?" Her rage over his racist remark bubbled over. "You and your Neanderthal tactics, Monty. Get a grip on yourself. A settlement could reduce our total expenses and get this matter off our agendas so we can focus on making money."

"I agree with Monty," Blackstone said. "We don't want to grasp defeat from the jaws of victory."

"You have a cliché for everything, Stan." Malouf's tone was unvarnished contempt.

"Without our specific approval, you had no right to offer to settle," said Pierce. "You have to withdraw any such directive today. Otherwise, Thanksgiving tomorrow will delay this almost a week."

"There is no offer, Monty. We are looking into a settlement. You're overreacting."

"If you screw up, you'll end up out of this big, plush office." His pale blues focused on her.

"Why don't you leave this plush office so I can get some work done?"

Blackstone and Pierce walked separate ways away from the corner suite.

Malouf struggled to find a way to motivate Hugh Harrison to drop the charges. A conviction of even a misdemeanor could have serious consequences for a physician. An hour later she got Attorney Jon Gullimore on the phone.

"Were you able to talk with Damjanovich?"

"We went back and forth a little. I think I could probably get them to take four hundred thousand today, maybe lower if we drag this out a while."

"And the assault charges are dropped?"

"No. That's just settling the contract disputes. Damjanovich said the figure to settle and drop the charge is seven figures. They know they have something you want."

"That's ridiculous."

"Consequences, Doctor. They're a bitch."

"My partners think we are close to winning the case. They want our legal fees extracted from Harrison."

"They're right about being close. The partial summary judgment was a huge help."

"I need the charge dropped, Jon," she sighed into the mouthpiece. "What do you suggest?"

"I recommend you talk that over with your defense counsel. It's going to be pricey if we include it with this negotiation."

"I just finished talking with a couple of the guys. They want you to go full tilt at winning and punish Harrison. I want to get rid of this stupid situation first."

"And they don't want to pay the price of your punch?"

"I never touched him."

"You don't need to spin your fiction to me, Dr. Malouf. Another solution is to pay Harrison personally, not out of Chandler."

"I'm not paying Harrison anything. End of story," Malouf hissed. "I need to think this through."

"A misdemeanor assault will be a black mark on your record. It may make it jeopardize your license and hospital privileges. It would be worth a hefty sum to get rid of this."

"Or just be found innocent."

"You should take the weekend and think this over. Give Harrison time to stew in his own juices, fitting for the season, I think." Jon Gullimore chuckled, apparently pleased with his humor.

Chapter 29

Thanksgiving

Inside the two-story contemporary Tudor home, Stacey and Stan Blackstone watched her parents and their daughter in the yard from the kitchen window. In the spacious kitchen, an artless blend of modern and traditional design, he was washing the large turkey broiler as she held an electric beater in an iced ceramic bowl full of whipping cream.

"I think the house needs to be in my name, Stan. Maybe jointly with my parents." She spoke with a Southern accent.

"I'm not going to lose this lawsuit, dear."

"Don't you have three going on? Isn't there a limit to how much the insurance company will pay out?"

"Yes. The maximum is one million per case and a total of three million for all claims."

"This poor woman's family is asking for thirty million. Don't that make you nervous?"

"Not in the least, Stace."

She shut off the beater. The room became quiet except for swishing of water in the sink and the gentle mechanical noise from the dishwasher.

"How can that be?"

"We have prayed about this. We'll be just fine."

"Maybe her family prays. Maybe the good Lord will favor them because they're poor and that little girl lost her mother."

"You've obviously not seen her family. The Lord guides the destiny of us all and he took her home. She's in a better place."

She sighed in frustration. "I'm just saying."

"Putting the house in your name would demonstrate a lack of faith."

"I think that faith is manifest in following God's will, not in being foolish."

"We shall be judged by our obedience to his laws but saved by grace. I'm depending on legal skill, the triumph of right and a little bit of grace."

"I just think it's foolish to risk the house and our savings like this, Stan."

"Did I tell you the home will be paid off in a couple of months?"

"The mortgage was over six hundred thousand. You couldn't possibly have made that much money."

"We owe about forty thousand. My year-end bonus will be at least that much." He toweled the pans dry.

"Has our income increased quite a bit over the last year or two?" She put the bowl on the counter with a clank, squinting and cocking her head.

"By the grace of God."

"I should pay more attention to the money." She retested the viscosity of the whipped cream with a spoon, then tasted her artistry. "So, Stan, how is it you make more money and work less time?"

"Remember the story of Jacob and Laban's sheep? We made a very good business deal."

"As I recall Jacob cheated Laban." She put the bowl in the refrigerator.

He knelt on a knee to put pans away in a low cabinet. When he straightened up, Stacey stood with folded arms and narrowed eyes. "You're not letting your love of money get in the way of salvation, are you, Stan?"

"I don't love money," he objected. "But, you have to admit, it is awfully nice to be so blessed."

She looked out the back window. Her parents were seconds away from the door. Rachel was hanging between them suspended by each arm.

"As long as it comes honestly."

Stan left to bring the port wine from the cabinet in their bedroom. Dessert was about to commence.

CHAPTER 30

The night before his scheduled mediation on Thompson's malpractice case Harrison went to bed but turned from side to side, front and back grappling with scenarios he might encounter in his defense. Speeches and responses played in various iterations many times over. Recollections of Sarah, his decisions, his logic and rationale cascaded as he adjusted his sheets and blankets searching for the tight temperature. He got out of bed in frustration at 2:30

in the morning. His house was cold. His thermometer displayed 17 outside. He padded into the kitchen to start the coffee.

He turned the heat up to seventy two, fired up a small space heater and put on sweatpants, sweatshirt, ski socks and a beanie. A tap on the keyboard brought the screen crackling to life. A spreadsheet with every point of data obtained during Sarah's hospitalization had been entered. He went to the closet and pulled out one of the large white poster boards he purchased for this occasion. Over the next hours he created color-coded graphs of blood pressure, heart rate, temperature, kidney function tests, ejection fractions and several blood tests. Other than ejection fraction, all the graphs were flat until Blackstone took over. On that date, the lines and the patient all went to hell.

With the graph complete and the coffee pot half empty, he looked at the Medline searches he had conducted on acute myocarditis. There were no studies even hinting at any medical therapy that altered mortality rate of patients with the disease. His search reconfirmed the use of dobutamine in heart failure led to increased mortality. The latter would not help him for two reasons. First, Jessop, instructed him not to comment on the care rendered by his partner because the liability company covered both Blackstone and him. They needed to prevail with both clients, a seemingly impossible task. Secondly, it would pit him against all the plaintiff's experts who supported using it despite the risk.

The phone rang at seven.

"Sam? How did you sleep?"

"Morning, Beth. I've been up a while."

"I have to be to work before nine. Would you like me to come over and fix you breakfast?"

"No. I'll be fine. I need to go over things and be prepared for this debacle."

"You're going to do great. Do you know what to expect?"

"Not really. I'm not sure of the format of the process."

"Hasn't your attorney filled you in?"

"Jessop hasn't said much. We meet at eight."

"Well, there goes breakfast anyway. You need to leave in half an hour."

"I do."

"Good luck, Hugh. Call me on my cell when you can."

"We'll see how it goes."

She sighed. "I missed you last night."

"I was not good company. We'll talk tonight."

The call ended. Harrison understood that many women wanted a rich cardiologist, even to the point of accepting one with many flaws. He no longer perceived himself as witty and debonair. After so much rejection and conflict he saw an unattractive, boring, introverted, emotionally detached old guy with impaired communication, affection and insight skills. His skin was lax, muscles small, teeth crowded, lips too thin, waist to fat and so on. He couldn't understand what Beth saw in him because she didn't need his money.

Jessop and Harrison sat in her office twenty minutes before the start of the negotiation. He wondered if she chose her attire based on whim or a purposed impression for her conflict of the day. Today, it was a power show, a deep red suit over a beige blouse, open at the neck with a plain gold cross on a short necklace and a white silk flower on the lapel.

"What is that?" She pointed at the papers in his hand.

"Here's a graph of all of Sarah Thompson's data when she was hospitalized."

"Let me see it."

He laid it on the walnut table in the small conference room. A list of dates ran across the top and every six hours ticked slightly below in black ink. Down the left side was a list of data in different colors of ink. The color-coded graph for each undulated slightly across most of the page before the lines abruptly diverted on Saturday and Sunday.

"This shows she was clinically stable all the time I took care of her."

"This might be interesting," Monica responded as she studied the large sheet. "Except for the fact that today we're not trying the case. We're seeing if we can agree on an amount of money that the liability company is willing to pay and that the multiple plaintiffs will agree to take. Each side will outline the merits of its position at the outset. Then we start to dicker. I don't think we'll need this today and I doubt Pope will let us use it if we go to trial. It hurts the case against Blackstone."

"Who is Pope?"

"Counsel for your insurance company, WIE."

"That makes it hard to defend myself. They're protecting themselves at my expense."

She shrugged. "I'm hired to defend you and I will."

He rubbed his neck and took a different tack. "How can you decide on a dollar amount without a thorough examination of the facts?

"The mediation process is short on facts and long on negotiation. Now, when we get there, I and Stan Henriod, Blackstone's counsel, will do all the talking. You should not offer anything except to answer questions if they come up. This is not an opportunity to try the case or lay out too many facts. If we try that, the mediation stalls and we'll get nowhere."

"That doesn't seem fair."

"That's the way it's done. If you feel compelled to say something, tell me first, Doctor. We can't afford to have statements blurted out, especially in front of the plaintiffs."

Harrison raised the sheets remaining in his hand. "I have two articles. One is from a textbook that says that Sarah's condition was one hundred percent fatal. The other is a paper from Europe that shows benefit from carvedilol treatment for acute myocarditis, the medication I gave."

She took the papers, glanced quickly at the top page and dropped it into her briefcase. "Don't blame Dr. Blackstone. Is that clear?"

"Won't say a word. Just look at the graph."

"We need to leave," she said.

He followed her for the five-minute walk to the office building of Hundley Hart. Again, they saw aluminum gulls in sculpted flight as they ascended in the glass-walled elevator. The corridor of the twelfth floor seemed dimmer, the painted names on the glass door, ominous. The oppressive hall held a small pride of lawyers. Blackstone stood out in his ill-fitting tweed sport coat and clashing patterned slacks. Harrison was no fashionista but most doctors were severely challenged when it came to dressing themselves.

Harrison did his best to relax as he knew these people in suits would be equally uncomfortable on his hospital turf. He tried to exude a sense of calm confidence.

"Hi, Monica," came from two of the men.

She returned the greeting and made introductions smoothly.

Franklin Pope, the attorney for the liability company, was trim and about six and a half feet tall with salt-and-pepper hair, impeccable suit, tortoise shell reading glasses and a clear tenor voice. "I think the best approach is to have one attorney from the three defendants make our statement. It should be reasonably short, just a few minutes. I asked Mike to prepare something, if that's all right with everyone else."

"As long he does a fair job of representing Dr. Harrison," Jessop said. "If not, I'll need a couple of minutes."

"We need to have a unified defense," Pope said. "We can't afford to have any blame shifted from one defendant to the other. Is everyone clear about that?"

"Dr. Blackstone got this whole mess started by an irresponsible and inflammatory remark," she pointed out.

"I did no s-such thing," Blackstone objected. When agitated he sometimes stuttered.

"For which, if he did, he is sorry," defended Henriod. "I'll represent all three parties without favoritism."

"I hope so," said Jessop. "Otherwise, I will speak."

"Talk to me first." Pope pointed a bony finger at her. The sharpness of his rebuke combined with the absence of interaction of any kind between the two cardiologists created a palpable tension.

"Let's get inside," Pope said and led the way.

Chapter 31

The group entered Hart's office. A young secretary trailing excessive floral scent brought them to the conference room. The mediator was an older Hispanic woman, looking out the window at the snow-covered peaks in the distance. She greeted the group and gingerly shook hands of those that knew her. Her knuckles were rheumatic. She directed the seating with attorneys at the table and the two doctors behind, against the wall.

Doug Thompson was dressed in a white shirt and skinny wrinkled tie. His hair was cut and combed back behind his ears, oiled in place. Ed Szabo sat next in line wearing a well-worn brown suit, decades out of vogue. To his left, Myra, in a bright Hawaiian muumuu, remained seated.

The mediator remained standing and addressed the group. "I'm Hazel Sanchez. I've practiced tort law well over twenty-five years. I'm a litigator by experience but started doing mediation about eight years ago. I've litigated 'med mal' as well as a variety of other corporate or business claims. Seeing the negative effects of prolonged conflict and capricious judgments, I came to appreciate the value of coming to agreements through other means. Two ways of settling differences outside of court include arbitration and mediation. In the former, a person or panel makes a judgment and the matter is settled. What we are doing today allows the parties to make a choice.

"We don't need to agree on anything today. None of the parties is bound to accept anything that is proposed but I expect you all to negotiate in good faith. So with that, let's start with introductions around the table, starting to my left with the plaintiffs and counsel."

Dennis Hart and another man were seated closest to Ms. Sanchez. He stood. "Dennis Hart, counsel for the four plaintiffs. This is Brett Ramussen, a new attorney in my firm. Next to me is Doug Thompson, father and guardian of Amy, the minor daughter of the decedent. Next are Myra and Ed Szabo—"

"Excuse me," Henriod interrupted. "Legal guardian?"

"Yes," Doug said.

"No," said Ed.

"The hell I'm not!" Doug said.

Ed folded his arms and rolled his eyes.

"What's going on?" Hart asked. "Do we need a minute?"

"No," Doug said. "We're all good."

"He's out on bail," Myra said. "We are the legal guardians."

"We became legal guardians when—"

"Bullshit! I'm her father, damn it. Jesus, Myra, get a—"

"Counselor, can you please get control?" Sanchez asked.

"We need a minute," Hart said.

"We'll step out," Pope said as he stood. "Let us know when you're ready."

All of the plaintiff squad left that room and went into an adjacent office.

"Well played," Pope said.

"It got interesting," Henriod said.

"We can't enter into an agreement with the girl unless the legal guardian does it," Pope said.

Ten minutes later, following some heated statements that the wall muffled, they were back in the room.

"As it turns out, Mr. Thompson is not the current legal custodian of the minor child but was when we filed and anticipates resuming that once the misunderstanding," Hart used air quotes, "is resolved. Since this is not a court proceeding, I ask your indulgence to allow him to remain here and involved."

Pope, Henriod, Jessop and Matt Parr, the attorney for the hospital, looked at each other and nodded agreement.

"Proceed," Sanchez said.

"Thank you. Let's see, this is Myra and Ed Szabo, parents of the deceased. They were partially financially dependent on her."

Ramussen, a stocky wrestler type, crewcut dirty blond hair, a scar over his left eyebrow and another on his chin, the look of a man who had seen conflict, said nothing.

After the plaintiffs and attorneys were identified, Sanchez spoke. "First Mr. Hart will present the complaint and allegations. Hopefully, it will take a few minutes to outline the most compelling arguments. While this is not a trial and the rules of the courtroom do not fully apply here, I expect respect, decorum and politeness." She looked directly at Doug.

"After all the presentations and questions and discussion, one group will leave the room. I will follow them, listen to their issues and come back here in a kind of shuttle diplomacy. If there are no questions, we'll proceed. Mr. Hart."

Ms. Sanchez took a seat, picked up a pen and positioned a yellow legal pad in front of her. Hart rested his elbows on the table, his large forearms, converged at the wrists. "But for the flagrant and possibly criminal negligence of these two cardiologists, we would not be here. Sarah Thompson would be raising her daughter and supporting her parents. Ignoring the emotional burden at the moment and looking at the financial loses only, her premature death resulted in a lifetime deficiency of over $5 million as was outlined in the complaint. People with her condition, myocarditis, often live decades with a transplanted heart. However, Sarah died in less than two weeks after her disease began without the benefit of timely referral to the experts who provide the type of care required for optimal management and survival. I call that callous disregard for her welfare for which she paid with her life. Her survivors are deprived of both her largess and the caring essence that characterized her life." Hart made a point of making eye contact with everyone on the plaintiff's side.

"If this case goes to court, we will show survival statistics of patients with acute myocarditis. We have three highly qualified expert witnesses from the best institutions in the United States, all of whom have already testified that the care rendered in the Olympus Center of Healing Arts for Sarah was substandard and contributed to her demise. Her impaired daughter will have lifelong financial needs that, if justice prevails, should fall upon the physicians and hospital that were negligent."

Hart referred to his papers. "Just to briefly review her course, she was admitted on Thursday, April thirteenth, to OCHA by Dr. Wallace Wren. The following day, a test showed her heart to be damaged and Dr. Harrison was consulted. He treated her with carvedilol, a medicine that, by the testimony of two of our heart failure experts, was inappropriate and contributed to her demise. This drug is known to decrease heart function and not approved for use in this condition anywhere in the world. Subsequently, each measure of her heart function showed deterioration. Her ejection fraction fell from 45 percent to 42 percent to 38 percent over a few days.

"Dr. Harrison failed to refer to a heart failure center, located in here in town. Heedless of her progressive deterioration, he did not substantively alter his ill-conceived regimen. By the time he left town on Friday, her function was down to 33 percent." He looked down his nose and angrily removed his thin reading glasses. He hurled the epithet, "33 percent."

He turreted to Blackstone. "To Dr. Blackstone's credit, he immediately recognized that Dr. Harrison had erred, based on a statement he made to the family. Nevertheless, he, too, failed to refer her to the heart failure center until she was near death. All of our experts have indicated that the use of dobutamine may have been appropriate but that the dosing was wrong." He looked over his reading glasses. "One wonders how patients survive in a hospital staffed with fools."

"Please, Mr. Hart," Sanchez interrupted, "be civil."

He barely paused. "By Sunday, Sarah was on full life support. Not until then was she was finally transferred to receive the treatment well past due. She died despite heroic efforts of the expert physicians and staff at Wasatch.

"There were many clear breaches of the standard of care resulting in the premature, unnecessary death of a young and successful mother. The fact of the matter is that the negligence manifest here borders on criminal. Her survivors have suffered catastrophic personal and financial losses because of the bad acts of the doctors and hospital. We intend to send a message that such incompetence will not be tolerated in our community or in our state."

Do they have courses every year in law school where they teach umbrage and righteous indignation, Harrison pondered as Hart fumed. *So full of himself, advocate for the underdog, the righter of wrongs, the warrior against evil and corruption.* What as ass. He watched Hart's clients through the diatribe. Doug dug at something under his fingernail. Ed's face was a mask. Myra blubbered, red eyes flowing, filling tissues.

"Thank you for your brevity, Mr. Hart," Sanchez stated. "Who is first for the defendants?"

"I'm speaking for all of us."

"Proceed, Mr. Henriod." She pronounced his name in three syllables as if it were Henry Odd.

"First, we are grieved that Sarah died at such a young age and difficult time. There is little any of us could say that would assuage your sorrow. As I lay out the defense of the physicians and hospital, it may be seem that they or we are indifferent to her contribution to you and to Amy. This is not the case. However logical it may seem to you to punish those you view as guilty of acts that led to her death, these are highly technical matters. Doctors go through at least four years of college and four years of medical school. Heart specialists spend another six years or more of training after graduation to acquire the skills and knowledge that allows them to successfully treat complex cardiac illness. That's fourteen years of study after high school, twice as long as it takes to practice law.

"This does not ensure that all physicians are excellent. There is a range of competence. Dr. Harrison has worked for close to twenty years in our community, built a successful and high-quality practice and recruited Dr. Blackstone into it. They are both highly esteemed in the medical community. It is felt by many, they are among the best cardiologists in our fair state."

His delivery was bland and he referred constantly to his notes with little eye contact with the people that mattered. Harrison was irritated that Jessop was not doing the talking.

"Myocarditis is a condition found in more than one percent of young to middle-aged adults who suffer accidental death from a variety of causes. Most of them presumably were asymptomatic and unimpaired. The condition goes away on its own. A tiny fraction has the aggressive form that results in progressive deterioration of heart function. Thousands of patients with this serious form have been studied with an array of medical treatments, none of which have been found to be superior to placebo or historic controls."

As Henriod droned, Doug lost interest and looked out the window.

"Carvedilol was approved for treatment of heart failure and has an impressive record of decreasing the chance of dying from it. Based on its favorable results, it is recommended as a first line drug in heart failure patients. Sarah had heart failure. To accuse someone of malpractice for using it for a generally approved indication is nonsense."

Doug startled, almost falling backward in his chair, hands flying up, releasing tiny particles of whatever he was mining from his nail beds. "Sorry," he said when he regained his balance.

It took Henriod a second to recapture his train of thought. "With respect to the failure to refer, Mrs. Thompson's vital signs had been stable until within about a day of her referral. Since there was no medical treatment proven to be effective in acute myocarditis, it was not unreasonable to treat her at the hospital near her family. The use of dobutamine by Dr. Blackstone is the standard of care for treating refractory heart failure. Even the experts for the plaintiffs testified to that fact. It is a non-issue.

"OCHA has both an excellent reputation and the outcomes data to support it. HealthMarks gives the hospital a five-point rating, the highest possible, in valve surgery, bypass surgery and in interventional cardiology whereas Wasatch has three-point rating in those same areas. Auspicious Healthcare, the owner of OCHA and scores of similar-sized hospitals, ranked it in the top 10 percent of its facilities. The objective data support it as a top hospital in cardiovascular treatment. In light of objective data and many awards, there is no basis for a claim against the facility. In addition, the complaint does not specify any act or omission that is in its purview. If it were derelict in allowing these physicians on staff, so were several other hospitals in the city. If any hospital excluded practitioners like these two well-qualified physicians, it would have no doctors on staff.

"As you know from our written response, we can and will provide data specific to the high level of expertise of these doctors as well as our own cardiology expert who will testify the care rendered by these men did not contribute to her demise. In the spirit of brevity offered by Mr. Hart, I will not dwell on these facts in evidence.

"While this may seem harsh, Sarah Thompson had a rapidly progressive disease, had good care in a top-of-the-line hospital and died regardless. A jury will find no fault. Again, our condolences to the family."

Stan took his place at the table, shuffling his papers into a leather folder. Otherwise, the room was silent for a moment. Mediator Sanchez was finishing her notes. Doug's chair rested with all for legs on the floor.

"Thank you," Hazel said. "Any questions?"

"Just to be clear," Hart said, "has the FDA approved carvedilol for myocarditis?"

"No," Henriod said.

"And there are no studies that show it to be either safe or effective in myocarditis, correct?" Hart said.

"Not to my knowledge," Henriod said.

"There is one small study that suggests both," Harrison said.

Henriod turned abruptly to Harrison, seated against the wall, not at the table.

"Here's an abstract of the study," Jessop said as she leafed through her briefcase.

After a few seconds she produced the piece of paper Hugh had handed her earlier. She slid it to Hart, who looked it over. The room went quiet.

"This is a tiny study and from Germany," he said.

The room stayed still.

Sanchez spoke. "If there's nothing else, Mr. Hart will take the Szabos and Mr. Thompson to another room now."

Hart stood and assisted Myra from her chair. Doug stood, dusting his hands on his new black cotton trousers.

"I'll join you in a minute after you've had a chance to converse," she told Hart. She waited until they were out of the room. "I'll be back here in fifteen to thirty minutes, hopefully not much longer than that. I know it's a slow process but that's how it is."

Harrison was disappointed that he had no opportunity to show his graph that had taken hours of insomnia to create. *Making a decision based on a few minutes of posturing and no objective information makes no sense to me*, he thought.

Far down the hall and through the closed door Doug could be faintly heard. "That was the biggest crock of shit I've ever heard."

"The process works best if the parties have their remarks filtered by the mediator," Sanchez said in response. "So, relax for a while." She left.

CHAPTER 32

Dennis Hart guided the coterie into a small library. "Can I get you anything? Coffee? Water? Soda?"

He told his secretary what to bring as they positioned around a table. Wooden chairs, not leather with adjustable height and rocking options, waited. Book bindings, acoustic tile and plush carpet absorbed sound. Recessed florescent lights shed a cool blue light. Three coffees entered. A bottled water went in front of Myra.

"These clowns don't have a case," Doug said. "I think this is just a tactic to delay the trial."

"A trial result is not a sure thing," Hart countered. "Juries can be funny. You hear of huge awards, like what we are asking, but they make the news because they are unusual. If we can get a high dollar amount today, that may well be better than what we could get at trial."

Doug poured some liquid from a worn silver and green flask into his coffee.

"A bird in the hand is worth two in the bush," Ed said.

"Birds, schmirds! These criminals need to suffer," Myra exclaimed. "They murdered our daughter. Jail would be too kind."

"They are going down," Doug said, gesturing like a rapper.

Ed hated everything about his former son-in-law and struggled to stifle the nearly uncontrollable urge to shut him up.

"Ms. Sanchez will want to leave here with a dollar figure as our first demand. The $30-million figure in our claim is going to be too high, that's for certain."

"Do we need to provide a lower number because we go first?" Ed asked.

Hart paused. "We could see what Ms. Sanchez says."

"What are you doing, Ed?" Myra twisted her upper body and her neck to look at him. They were on the same side of the table with Doug opposite.

"Asking a question."

"Let's start with $50 million," Doug said.

"Couldn't they be charged with a crime? Manslaughter, negligent homicide or reckless endangerment or something." Myra wanted blood and had been watching *Law & Order* reruns on cable.

"That's up to the district attorney. There's no money in that for you. Besides, if they're in jail, they have no income," Hart explained.

"I know a little bit about criminal law," Doug offered.

"Yeah. How to get caught," Ed said.

"Smart ass."

"We already have a number on the table," Ed said. "It's in the complaint supported with rationale. Let them explain why a lower offer is more fair. Never be the first to put up a figure."

"What do you know?" Myra asked. "Just shut up and sit there."

Ed was almost immune the insults. Almost. He thought about wringing her neck.

There was a knock. Ramussen opened the door. Hazel Sanchez lumbered in. Sitting in the chair at the head of the table she grimaced. "Arthritis," she said. She placed the yellow pad in front of her and pulled to page three or four. She then rested her hands in front of her, fingers deviated away from her thumbs on both hands. "You may speak freely in front of me. I don't tell the other side what you say but I convey how you feel in the most effective way I can to get to an agreement. When I leave this room, I want to bring them a demand in dollars. So, what did you think about the defense?"

"You have a figure in the amended complaint," Ed said. "Thirty million dollars. I think it would be best if you went to their room now and asked for a response to that."

"It'll go nowhere," she said. "The doctors will not approve because it exceeds the payment limits of their insurance policies. They would need to pay from their personal assets."

"And they should," Myra said.

"Let them propose something else, an amount they can defend. My clients are talking about bringing a criminal complaint against the physicians."

"Damn right," Doug said.

"They're angry with the delays imposed by the process."

"Amen," he said.

"And need the money to care for this little Down syndrome girl."

"What can I offer them?" Sanchez asked. "It would speed things up if I have a dollar figure from you."

"If their offer is good, we'll forego the criminal complaint," Dennis said. "If their total offer is not over $5 million, we'll pick up our marbles and go home. It is a virtual certainty we will get that much at trial, given the strength of our case."

Ed cleared his throat to let Hart know he was displeased.

"That sounds like a number to me," Sanchez said.

"I'm not interested in delaying the inevitable and getting more billable hours as the defense attorneys do. I cannot waste my resources." Hart was righteous. "So, go. Tell them the first response to our claim is theirs."

"What do you think?" Ed asked Ramussen.

"I'd up the ante to thirty-one million. Then the bastards will know that we're not in a negotiating mood over here."

"I like this young man," Myra said.

"Brett is new to this," Hart said. "But, if they want a figure, go with that for starters."

"Not $5 million? You want to shut this process down before it starts?" Sanchez asked.

Hart waved her out the door. She lumbered out.

"What if the statute of limitations has expired?" Ed said. "It may be too late to charge them in criminal court."

"What do you mean too late?" Myra demanded.

A round of argument then ensued.

In the conference room on the other side of the office there was laughter.

"I think I can beat that. You remember the case I defended last year," Stan Henriod said to the attorneys for the hospital and the insurance company. "This fifty-year-old scheduler at a trucking company was burned out. She had three mechanical heart valves. She moaned about her life, how her husband had retired and that she wanted to travel with him. In order to do so, she needed to have income, such as complete disability. Her doc would only give her a partial rating. So, she decreased her anticoagulation dose, hoping for a minor little something to happen. It did. She had a small stroke then sued for mismanaging her anticoagulation. How do people think they can get away with this stuff?"

"We just had a case where a cardiologist north of here was sued for a stress-test report," Jessop countered. "He read the test as mildly abnormal but low risk and faxed a handwritten report, which was in the records of the referring doctor. The typed report followed. Four years later the patient died of a heart attack. Four years! The family sued the primary doctor, claiming he should have done more, like referring the guy to a cardiologist. They also sued the cardiologist, who had never seen the patient except for a few minutes during the stress test."

"Abnormal stress test? Should have done an angiogram," Blackstone said.

"Not according to guidelines and data," Harrison said.

"Not the best case to bring up, Monica," Pope said.

A knock was followed by the door opening. Everyone looked at a watch as Sanchez came in and eased into a soft chair. "That didn't take too long, now did it?" She opened her yellow pad. "You have an angry group in the other room. They are openly hostile and would prefer to bring this case into the criminal courts. I think their attorney has his hands full trying to prevent that from happening."

"Criminal?" Pope said. "Oh, come now. That's patently ridiculous."

"I'm not implying they have a case," Hazel said calmly. "I'm just letting you know about their state of mind."

"Did they come up with a number?" Pope asked the question as he rocked back and forth in his chair.

"First they said there is a number in the complaint. Then they said thirty-one million. It's your job to counter."

No one spoke for a while.

"Do they have a specific animus? Henriod asked. "I guess what I want to know is does the award get split equally three ways."

"Everything is on the table," Sanchez answered. "They said they are willing to forego the criminal charges if the settlement is high enough."

Blackstone tapped Henriod on the shoulder and asked, "Criminal charges, as in going to jail?"

He nodded.

"I did nothing wrong," Blackstone whined. "Everyone knows that Harrison killed the girl."

Harrison gasped exasperation.

"What kind of an egotistical ass are you?" Jessop asked loudly. "Have you looked at the data? Where is that graph?" She ripped out Hugh's handmade poster. "Look at this!" She tapped angrily on the place where the lines all went down. "If a jury sees this graph and how stable the patient was until you assumed her care, you will not look innocent."

He looked closely.

She continued. "As far as I know, you both did the best you could. But don't think for a minute you couldn't lose everything you own. Look at those lines! A jury would eat them up."

Blackstone's face sagged, his color drained.

Jessop went on. "If you truly believe that Dr. Harrison's treatment resulted in her death, I, I...." She felt Sanchez's gaze and sat angrily in her chair. "I don't have words for this."

"Mrs. Thompson had giant cell myocarditis," Harrison said. "It is one hundred percent fatal. No one survives it without a heart transplant." He waved an article he had copied. "No one in the world has an effective medical treatment. A reasonable jury, once they hear that, they will be inclined to think the family is simply out to get rich."

"Can you excuse us for a minute?" Henriod asked Sanchez. "We need to confer in private."

After she left, Henriod spoke. "You have the checkbook, Frank. What are your thoughts?"

"I think Dr. Blackstone needs a break. You can't say stuff like that in front of the negotiator, Doctor."

Blackstone rolled his eyes. "She's not judge or jury."

"I'm serious, Dr. Blackstone. What you just did harmed your defense, believe it or not."

"Truth is the best defense. The truth is that he killed the patient."

Franklin Pope sighed. "Well, Doctor, you are welcome to your own opinion. It harms you and everyone else when you voice it like that. Take a walk and think about that for a few minutes."

"Let's take a break in the hall," Henriod said.

He took a few steps toward the exit. Blackstone didn't move.

"Please," Parr said, breaking his silence.

Blackstone left with his attorney.

When the door closed, Pope asked, "Is he always like this?"

"I'd almost forgotten how annoying he can be," Harrison said.

"Your statement was excellent, Dr. Harrison. I think Hazel will think long and hard about that."

"What do you think we should offer, Frank?" Jessop asked.

"Sixty thousand total. That's twenty for each defendant. Whoever sees it will recognize it was a frivolous claim and settled to get rid of the nuisance."

"That's good with me," said Parr.

"Don't you have a son in an Ivy League school back East, Frank?" Jessop asked.

The conversation turned to passing time until Henriod returned with his grumbling, disgruntled client a few minutes later. Hazel Sanchez followed them in and restarted the process.

"It doesn't appear that they are serious," Pope said. "We would prefer that they produce a number far less than the claim, but, for the sake of moving things along, we will offer sixty thousand total for all respondents."

"They'll say that's ridiculous," Sanchez said.

"It's more than they deserve," Jessop responded. "You heard the doctor. She died of an untreatable, one hundred percent fatal disease. Here it is, in print." Monica pushed the article to her across the table. "We have a decent chance of skating at trial."

"You're going to make me earn my fee, I can tell." She limped out.

"If the death of a young mother comes to a jury," Harrison said, "and they see her kid with Down syndrome every day, the facts get lost in the emotion."

"Which is exactly why we're here," Pope said.

"Right will prevail," Blackstone said.

"That would make me very nervous, if I were you," Jessop said, pointing again at the graph.

"Don't get him started," Pope said.

Harrison chuckled. Blackstone began a rant about his superior education and accomplishments.

CHAPTER 33

A few minutes later, after time to construct her approach, Sanchez entered the library where Hart watched Doug simmer in anger. Myra sipped on her water. Ed read an old magazine.

"This is a slow process," Sanchez said. "I get the feeling it's going to take a while." She sat and peeled through pages on her yellow legal pad, licking her thumb in the process. "They were unhappy with your decision to stick with the figure in the complaint. They don't think you're serious about the mediation."

"I'm not very excited about it either," Myra said. "We're going to get cheated."

"They gave me a low number, so low that you may be outraged. Don't be. Realize we need to start somewhere." She looked at the three petitioners.

Ed looked at her over the crumpled pages of the newspaper he held. He saw a page of doodles in front of Doug. The table was clean before Myra. She was the only one there not bored by doing nothing except staring into space.

"What did they say?" Hart asked.

"They said that Sarah had an incurable form of the disease, a hundred percent fatal, no known effective medical treatment." She let the copy of the article float down in front of Hart.

"I'm not in the mood for spin," Hart said kindly but firmly. "We have three experts that agree she was horribly mismanaged. We can easily get more. What was the figure they offered?"

"Sixty thousand."

"Ha!" he roared. "For each? Unbelievable!"

Hart was at his indignant best and Ed found it entertaining. A slight smile emerged.

"Total. It's just a starting position. It might have been higher had you provided a figure lower than thirty million. All it means is that they do not want to pay millions of dollars. It's understandable."

"We're finished then. I have spent more than that just to get to this point," Hart said.

"They screwed up!" Myra yelled. "They know it and they need to pay for it."

Doug muttered an epithet, accusing them of incestuous behavior.

"I have to admit it's a bold move when they don't have a snowball's chance in hell of winning," Hart said.

"They think they have a good chance," Hazel observed in a neutral tone.

"Sarah would be alive today if they had just referred her sooner, before she was already dead."

"They say her disease," she looked at her notepad, "is one hundred percent fatal. Obviously, I know nothing about that but that is their position." She pointed at the paper in front of Hart. He studied it quickly.

"Fatal without a transplant and that's the point. Let them use this article as it works in our favor."

"It's bullshit," Doug said. "Why haven't we heard that until today?"

"Good question," said Hart. "It could be a bluff. No one is under oath today. Hold on."

He left with the paper in hand. Ed wanted to read it but, knowing there would be a lot of time and boredom ahead, said nothing.

"They lie like a rug," Doug said. "Greedy sons of bitches." He went to the window and muttered, "God knows I could use some real money right now."

"It's Amy's money," Myra said. "Not yours."

He turned to face her. "I'm her parent. It'll go to me."

"It'll go to a trust fund," Ed said. "That's how this works. You'll draw from the fund for her needs."

"Ed, you should just shut up," Myra said. "You like to think you're a know-it-all and really you don't know diddly."

"So, you think money for Amy will go to Doug with no conditions?" Ed argued.

"You're right, Mr. Szabo," Ramussen said. "Typically awards for minors and the disabled go into a trust account with a professional that manages the funds and disperses them according to the financial needs of the awardee."

Doug cursed again. The door opened and Hart reentered.

"I asked my secretary to do a search on the giant cell issue. That'll take a few minutes."

"Why don't we just cut our demand to $6 million and see how they respond," Ed said.

"Who made you the negotiator, Ed?" Myra shot. "Let the lawyers do what they do. That doctor killed my daughter and I don't care what it takes, I'm going to make him suffer." Myra pushed away from the table and began to rock back and forth in her process to stand. She came to her feet. "Dr. Harrison should not have a license to practice medicine. He should be in jail. I wonder how many other young women have died at his hand." Her face grew crimson. "The hospital should have kicked him out. His old group had the good sense to, right after Sarah died. The hospital sweeps these inconvenient deaths under the rug and keeps making money hand over fist. I looked at their public reports. They made over four million dollars the year they slaughtered my daughter." She began to cry in earnest. "Oh, God. It's not fair. It's not right. They can't get away with it. I won't let them." She leaned her back heavily against the wall, sobbing.

"Neither will I," Hart said.

"A mediation is not about justice," Ed stated. "It's about money."

"I want justice!" she shrieked.

"This is in civil court, not criminal," Ed said. "You want justice, file charges."

"I think I will."

"How appropriate that one of the attorneys is named hemorrhoid? Righteous! Anyways, we get nothing if the law puts them in jail. What we want is to siphon their money for the next thirty years into our wallets. And it's legal if we use lawyers to fight for us," he pointed at Hart and Ramussen. "We stay out of the big house."

Sanchez groaned.

"And who made you a philosopher?" Myra now pointed her finger at him, wagging it back and forth. "The money goes to Amy, you—"

"Easy, easy," Hart pled. "Let's get back on track. There may be some merit in doing what Ed suggested. We'll learn a lot from their response."

"I think it's a reasonable step," echoed Sanchez. "In these mediations, if there is no movement toward some mid-point, they stalemate."

"I'd suggest we go to twenty million," Hart said. "I don't want to give up too much ground too fast. I'd like to see the internet search but first it will take a while to find and print the information and it'll take a while to decipher and digest it. Going down and testing their ability to compromise while we assess this other issue is good. What do you think?"

"If we take a big step down and they make a tiny step up, we know we're done," Ed said.

Doug shrugged.

Myra objected. "No. Go down maybe one million, not ten. I don't care what any of you think, it's not just about money."

"I know you're upset, Mrs. Szabo," said Sanchez. "God knows, you ought to be. Too little of a drop will stall or stop the process. If you are interested in getting money for certain and soon, your demand must go down so their offer will go up."

"Let's make a deal!" Doug mimicked.

"Shut your trap, Doug," Myra yelled. She wavered as she stood with her hands on the back of her chair, then sat.

"Six million will tell us if they will budge much," Ed said. "Twenty or thirty won't tell us a thing."

"You are an idiot," Myra said.

"He has a point," Ramussen said.

Hart glared at him.

"Will that speed things up?" Doug asked.

"It certainly will," Sanchez said.

"I really want to get this settled today," Doug said.

"I don't care what you want," Myra said.

"We're not going to get twenty million or ten million or even six today," Ed said. "We just need to know how much they'll move."

"How do you know so much, Mr. Smartypants?"

"We see lawsuits at work. And I have been known to read the paper."

"You should just sit there, be seen and not heard." Myra pointed her chubby finger at Ed. "You are going to screw this up. The both of yous."

"So, Dennis, what do you want me to tell the other room?" Sanchez asked.

"Let's go with ten million."

"No," Myra said.

"Fine," said Doug.

"Go ahead," Ed shrugged.

Sanchez left. The door closed. Myra seethed.

"How much weight have you put on since Sarah died?" Doug spat out. "Are you trying to eat yourself to death?"

"Doug," Hart said, "that's not helpful. Let's take a walk."

"I mean, you've always been fat, but now you are huge. Damn. And I had forgotten just how pleasant it is to be around you."

Hart pulled at his shoulder. Doug twisted away.

"Full of nice things to say about Ed and me and anyone else who happens to fall within your huge gravitational field." He gestured broadly with both tattooed arms. His face gleamed with enjoyment. "You are so soft and cuddly for ol' Ed there. Oh, baby!"

"You're a leech," Myra exploded, red in the face. "You never contributed to Sarah's life except to give her a defective child. She paid alimony to you, you miserable excuse for a man!"

"Doug, please!" Hart pled. "You need a break."

Myra stood. Her hands supported her on the table. Doug sat down on a wood chair, pushed back, balancing on the hind legs, his feet on the table. "What, Myra? Are you going to sit on me? Death by ASS-fixiation." He laughed loudly as he put his feet on the floor and all chair legs down. "I'll charge you with ASS-ault." He roared with mirth, tossing his long hair.

"Myra, let's go out for a minute," Hart said, moving in her direction.

"You are disgusting!" She pointed at Doug, red in the face, trembling.

She tried to move away from the table but staggered. Ed and Hart rushed to support her but was too late. She caught her foot and fell, slamming into the floor with a shudder. Her eyes went wide as they all heard a snap.

"Oh. My hip." Then she screamed.

"Can you get up?" Hart asked.

"Oh, my hip!" she replied. "Oh, God." Her arms flailed and her color went sallow.

"Brett, call an ambulance," Hart said.

Ramussen left.

"He pushed me," Myra howled.

"Everyone saw what happened," Ed said.

"He attacked me. My God, it hurts."

Doug left the room. Hart fussed around Myra, trying to figure out how to make her more comfortable but every time he touched her she cried out.

"Oh, it hurts! Oh God, oh God. Help me, Ed, dammit."

"Ten million," said Sanchez after a full minute of verbal tap dance in the conference room.

"That's a healthy drop," Jessop said. "Lopped 66 percent off."

"It's still totally unrealistic for a settlement," said Henriod. "Where is Hart in all this? Is that his number?"

"The bigger the award, the more for him and his firm," offered Pope.

"His figure was higher but the family there is all over the map," Sanchez said.

"This might be a lot easier if there were only one plaintiff," Jessop said.

"Sarah was financially supporting her parents," Henriod said. "They lost that income and they provide a lot of care for Amy."

"They got life insurance for that," said Blackstone.

"They came down by two thirds. We should go up by a third," Pope offered.

"Less than a hundred thousand?" Sanchez asked. "This will end there if that's your figure. They are looking for a big increment."

"Excrement," said Blackstone. "They're full of it."

"Do you have an upper limit?" Sanchez asked of Pope.

"One absolute limit," Jessop replied, "is that the award, if any, must be less than the policy limits. That is one million dollars for each physician. My guess is that Frank will have a much lower limit."

"You're right," he said.

"What is it?" Sanchez asked.

"I'm not going to say."

"Ninety K," Henriod said. "Propose thirty from each of us." He looked around for support and found only one nod and that was from Frank Pope.

"You can propose ninety if you want," said Blackstone, "but none of it's from me. I did nothing wrong. I'm not going to pay a nickel and I'm not going to have some malpractice payment on my record for the rest of my life."

"You've already got three," Henriod said. "And you've two more in the barrel besides this one."

"Which is exactly why I can't let this frivolous suit succeed."

"Just say ninety thousand," Jessop said. "We'll iron out the attribution if they accept it."

Sanchez left.

"How many losses until you find someone is uninsurable?" Harrison asked Pope.

"Three in a decade."

Harrison raised his eyebrows. Pope maintained a blank face.

"You're still insuring me," Blackstone said.

"Against my better judgement," Pope said.

The door opened a moment later. Sanchez walked in.

"They like it. It's accepted."

Shock spread around the room.

"I'm kidding. Mrs. Szabo fell and hurt her hip. They've called the paramedics. This session is over."

"Does she need a doctor?" Harrison asked.

"She certainly does," Sanchez said. She smiled. "Anyone but you. She'll survive until the ambulance crew arrives."

Chapter 34

April 2007

Heel clacks reverberated in the Marchetti Building as Jennifer Hayes and Sarisha Malouf coincidentally entered the echoic hall about the same time from different directions. They exchanged cool greeting and made their way into a small office adjacent to the OCHA boardroom.

"Thanks for coming on short notice," Zone uttered. "Mindy is on her way."

"Mindy? Who is that?" Malouf asked.

"I thought you knew, Sarisha," Zone answered, sipping from a black, cylindrical ceramic. "Chad left a few months ago. Mindy is our new chief financial officer."

"It's a good thing that the assault charge against you was dropped," Hayes said with a smirk.

"The county attorney wanted a case he could win. With no evidence, they had no case."

"Harrison lost his leverage in your legal tangle."

"He sure did."

"So you haven't settled with him yet?" Jennifer, the nosy, annoying woman, asked.

"No. If any of our docs even dreams about breaking one of their agreements, I'll punish them."

"Any problems with the cardiac cath lab agreement from your perspective?" Hayes asked.

"It's working well."

It has probably increased everyone's income by 50 to 100 percent, so it ought to be working well, Hayes thought.

Mindy hurried in. She had a solid muscular body, brown hair and thick eyebrows behind glasses. She carried a small stack of books and Liles. "Hi, everyone. Hope I didn't keep you waiting." Her voice was mousy, nasal and Minnesotan.

Zone shifted and cleared his throat. "There may be a problem with the cath lab contract, Sarisha. I got a call about it this week from a friend of a friend, so to speak. Someone in the U.S. Attorney's office has it on their radar. It makes me a little nervous."

"Our attorney said it's clean."

"Our attorney is also confident. Has anyone called you or your clinic manager to ask about it?"

"I haven't spoken to anyone."

"If you get a call, don't give out any information," Zone continued. "If an attorney calls, refer them to us or to your own legal folks."

"I spoke with Bill, your practice manager," Hayes added. "I gave him the same message this morning."

Zone tag-teamed the conversation. "Our counsel asked us to run a projection of the financial impact of dismantling the arrangement, in case it comes to that."

"We have two years almost before the automatic renewal."

"There are provisions for early termination if certain criteria are met."

A sheet of dollar signs and figures slid in front of each of them and a discussion ensued that tugged hard at Malouf's digestive tract. When she pulled his eyes away from the figures, she noted that Hayes was looking out the window with a slight smile on her face. The bitch was enjoying this.

"This is all an unnecessary exercise. There's nothing legally questionable about what we're doing."

"We have to have a contingency in place for this threat."

"Potential threat," Malouf corrected, not believing a single word from his skinny, lying lips. She stood to leave. "Life is full of them. Sounds more like a rumor."

"I just needed to let you know."

"Now I know. Anything else?"

"Nothing urgent."

"Good. I'm heading downtown for another tangle with Harrison."

Can't trust administrators, Malouf thought as she left. *Duplicity and mendacity seemed to be required traits to work in hospital administration. When they need you, when they're on your side, life is good.*

She went straight to the office then down to the entrance where Bruce, a young receptionist at Chandler Cardiovascular pulled up driving her silver Mercedes. She climbed in the back seat, squeezed his muscular shoulder and sat back in irritation.

She knew the reason for cath lab contract was one of several blows intended to kill St. Lucius Hospital. The strategy worked. It had gone out of business and the building sold to a software firm. But this reason had not been part of the language of the agreement so as far as she knew they had no reason to worry. But now OCHA might want to end the contract out of some lame, imaginary excuse. "U. S. Attorney's Office, my ass," she muttered.

"Beg your pardon, Doctor. Did you say something?" Bruce looked through the rearview mirror.

"Not to you, Bruce."

Malouf made a couple of phone calls and didn't speak at all to the kid during this drive. He dropped her off at the Boston Building entrance in a ripping gust. He drove away as she hurried to shelter in another marble foyer.

Up the elevator and off on the seventh floor she found a group of familiar figures and faces huddled outside the office of Christianson and King, where three previous sessions had been held over the last month. Her partners were in uniform, she thought, mismatched sport coats and slacks. Pierce, hair bushy and wild, his walrus mustache in full bloom, approached. "I hope this was not a mistake," was his greeting.

"The judge almost forced us to go this route," she answered.

"Dr. Malouf," Gullimore greeted as he approached.

"Counselor," she said with a smile.

"I hope this was not a mistake," he said.

"We'll know later today," she said.

"Arbitrators tend to cut the baby in half," he said. "I think we would win everything in court."

"You're the one who had to buy off on this," Pierce said.

"I was afraid the judge would be offended if we failed to take his recommendation. As it turned out, he had just returned from a week long seminar on arbitration and alternative dispute resolution."

"So, what happens today?" Pierce asked.

By now all four of the partners surrounded her and Gullimore.

"He's mostly made his decision. He wants both sides to summarize, however, before he finalizes his findings. He wants to hear what we have to say, spend an hour or two for last minute fine tuning then announce."

The door to the office opened and the crowd flooded in. The elevator door opened and Damjanovich and Harrison exited and followed the crowd.

A few minutes later Damjanovich painted a picture of a near saintly Harrison and evil partners. Harrison had complied with the contract, given his required notice of departure and fulfilled his part of the agreement written in plain English including one of the two non-competition clauses. The other clause was clearly an oversight by the careless attorney who wrote it. He deserved his money. He droned one. Sarisha thought of him as an anesthesiologist attorney, one that put everyone to sleep. Harrison sat there, bending his little finger over and over, wincing every now and then, probably trying to restore his range of motion.

"Plain English," said Jon Gullimore when it was his turn. "Read the contract. It is crystal clear. If Dr. Harrison practiced in competition with Chandler Cardiovascular, he was to forfeit his accounts receivable and deferred compensation. No matter how fair or not anyone might think that is, all the cardiologists signed agreements with this exact language. It doesn't matter that he founded the group. Everyone had to play by the same rules. He didn't. He competed when he joined the Pioneer Heart Institute and thereby forfeited his money." Gullimore was indignant when he emphasized, "Plain, clear, concise, unequivocal, his claim is baseless. Ours is fully supported."

Malouf was very pleased. She followed Damjanovich as the courtroom emptied. Country club and cigar bar attitude simmered beneath Leo's wool worsted pinstripes. His boney fingers massaged the resting place high on the long, straight Ibizan hound nose under his tortoise shell glasses. He pulled Harrison aside. She had to pass by. She went to the elevator as they chatted.

Harrison watched Damjanovich enter the elevator with Sarisha and crowd, checked his watch, then walked with purpose to the stairway. A few buildings away he entered the office of the U. S. Attorney.

Seated and waiting in an atrium outside the elevator were three well-dressed people, two women and a man.

The man studied Harrison as he exited the closing doors. "Dr. Harrison?"

"Yes. Are you Mr. Dominici?"

"Joe Dominici," he said as he and the women stood. He extended his hand. "I'm surprised to find you here," he said as they shook. "These are my associates from Higgins Cowen here with me. Lisa Jacobs and Monica Moynihan."

They greeted him with handshakes.

"This is Dr. Hugh Harrison."

The whistleblower attorneys said they were pleased to meet him.

"I recognized you from your photo," Joe Dominici said.

"I'm glad I caught you. I had a break and came here in the off chance we could meet. Your email indicated you had an appointment at eleven."

"This meeting is crucial," Dominici explained. "If Swift, the U.S. Attorney, is not interested in pursuing this matter, it becomes a steep uphill battle with only a small chance of success. We would choose not to represent you."

"Could you meet us for lunch, Doctor?" Jacobs asked. "I'm sure this meeting will not take long."

"I have a conflict at one."

"I'll call you when we're done here," Dominici said.

"Mr. Swift will see you now," the receptionist announced, pointing down a hall to her right.

"Should I go in with you?" Harrison asked.

"Not this time," Dominici said.

They entered the office.

Harrison now had almost two hours to kill. Christianson wanted to deliver his decision in a meeting where he could see both parties.

Chapter 35

Back on the street in the crowd and sunlight, Hugh bumbled along with nowhere to go. He passed a tobacco store where he bought half a dozen cheap Prince Edwards, his grandfather's preference. He hadn't smoked much after age twenty-five and then only cigars.

He strolled past the Salt Lake City and County building where his great-grandfather, a Mason, had set five stories of stone. A few minutes later he saw sallow Ed Szabo entering an office building together with a woman. He held the door for her as she entered turning, nodding, smiling. Ed's face bore no expression as usual.

It was almost exactly noon when his phone rumbled. Joe Dominici and associates were looking for lunch recommendations. He met up with them a few minutes later.

"Dr. Harrison, we may have something here," Dominici said as they battled the midday press. "Pete Swift, the U. S. attorney, sounded interested in very general terms. We omitted specifics but the hypotheticals and generalities seemed to intrigue him."

He gave an overlong account of the conversation. The Second Street Grill was busy and looked full but they did not need to wait long for a table.

Idle chatter occupied time until a server in a white shirt and black apron took their orders. "Monica," Dominici said, "tell the good doctor what you think."

"Whistleblower cases are notoriously difficult. As you probably know, Dr. Harrison, there are few firms that are successful in this area. The key is in case selection. It is paramount that the United States Attorney with jurisdiction has an interest in pursuing the case. These lawmen are usually only interested if the government has lost a lot of money and if the entity has deep pockets so they can recover the losses and add penalties and interest. They like cases that are easy to prove, flagrant abuses. If the behavior is marginally over the legal line, they don't pursue it. High profile cases, you know, career-enhancers, get priority."

Harrison was distracted by her facial asymmetry as she talked and looked away so he could listen better.

"They like informants that are reliable, without a criminal history and preferably professional and credible. For example, we described you as an esteemed local physician with an outstanding reputation. We also said your knowledge was true insider information, not publicly available. The losses to Medicare alone we put at four or five million, not a big number. On the other hand, it seems to be a breach of the consent decree and that's a huge fine. Swift, the attorney, is young and upwardly mobile. I think he'd love to nail both a corrupt national corporation and a bunch of greedy physicians." She faced Dominici. "At least, that's how I read his response."

Rather than respond verbally, Dominici looked at Jacobs for her response.

"I didn't detect as much enthusiasm as I did caution," Jacobs said. "I agree that he's interested."

Dominici nodded. "Which is huge. If these cautious yet ambitious prosecutors see blood in the water, they go aggressive. I'd like to set a deadline for building your case, Dr. Harrison and when we have it solid, make an appointment with Mr. Swift again and lay it out in detail."

"Just tell me what to do."

"I'm going to have Lisa work with you on your affidavit. We have a copy of the contract at issue. That is key."

"Are you sure you can use it?" Hugh asked. "It's protected by a court order, only to be used with respect to that claim."

"It's restricted to a claim you have regarding Chandler Cardiovascular, which this is," Moynihan said. "At least, we're going to push to include them so that this document won't be excluded."

"We can subpoena the contract. If they try to pull a fast one, we have your copy for comparison," Dominici added. "Is it possible for you to get actual financial data about the amounts of money Medicare and all government agencies have paid for patients covered by the contract?"

"No. I have nothing about finances."

"That would be helpful but not critical," Dominici said. "We showed Swift some portions of the consent decree between the Justice Department and Auspicious Healthcare. I thought we got his attention with the breaches you believe they committed."

"Yeah, I thought so, too," Moynihan said. "Breaking the decree is both a civil breach and a criminal act. The fines could be enormous."

"What about the hospital that went under? Our Lady of Something," Lisa said. "Do they know about this agreement?"

"Saint Lucius. I told them in general terms a few years ago. They ignored it."

"They have incurred a large loss in part because of it. It surprises me they didn't give it more attention."

"This was just one of several things that Auspicious did to compete."

"Who owned Saint Lucius?"

"Pacific Hospital Group."

"Really? They're based in L.A. I know a couple of attorneys in their office."

At ten to one Hugh left for the Christianson King office.

An hour later Harrison walked slowly with Damjanovich back to his nearby office. They were speechless.

Once they got inside his building Leo said, "I've never seen or heard of an arbitration that turned out so lopsided."

"Stock, deferred compensation and accounts receivable, they're all gone," Hugh said.

Leo had nothing to say.

"Add to that the $300 thousand I've already paid you and almost half a million dollars to pay their legal expenses. Close to two million bucks, net loss."

"I can't believe he did that."

"I'm looking for work, Leo. I don't have $500 thousand, even if I sell my house. I'm screwed."

"There must be hundreds of jobs for a good cardiologist."

"None of the groups around her is interested in hiring me. The Veterans Hospital and University are not hiring. It would take half a million dollars to start up another solo practice and even if I had the money, the prospect of doing that is unattractive not to mention risky."

"You'll find something."

"I have a short locum tenens job in Arizona later this month."

"A temporary job?"

"A three-week gig."

"Well, that's something."

"How am I going to pay them?"

"I'll try to arrange payments over, what, five years?"

"And if they want it now?"

"How much equity is in your home?"

"My home equity tanked like every other house. It's less than fifty thousand. Not even a tenth of what I owe."

"I'll work something out, Doctor."

They arrived at the door with sandblasted glass and a *Dingle & Damjanovich* sign in black paint. Leo opened and they both entered. His secretary, a fifty-something woman nodded and smiled.

"Without a steady job, I have no way to pay June," Hugh said.

"June?"

"My ex."

"You should seek a modification of alimony."

"That's in progress. I meet with my divorce attorney tomorrow. Which I can no longer afford."

"What other assets do you have?"

"Negligible," he said. "I never should have sued the bastards. It came back to bite me hard."

"Why don't you go back to work with that other group, whatever they're called."

"Pioneer Heart. My accountant pointed out I'd be on the hook for about two million for a required buy back when a couple of stock holders leave or retire. I don't need more debt."

"Isn't there another group in town?"

"Like I said, no one will touch me."

"I'm sorry, Doctor."

"It's not your fault, Leo. It's just how things have turned out." Harrison stood by the door, not wanting to sit or stay.

"Let me get your parking validated."

Harrison pulled out into traffic and headed home. The thought of facing Beth made him shudder. Instead of taking the off-ramp to his house, he kept driving, heading to a nearby canyon, where he could try to wrap his mind around his predicament.

CHAPTER 36

Ed came in the side door with a paper sack of groceries and Amy following behind.

"We're home," he proclaimed.

"So am I," came the terse reply from the front room.

"Hi, Grandma."

"Don't trip on the oxygen, honey."

After placing the food on the chipped tile counter, he came to check on his wife. "It's good to see you up, Myra."

Myra moved slowly behind an aluminum walker, tethered by a light green tube that wrapped around her ears and ended in prongs up her nose. "Did you pick up my prescriptions?"

"I did. How was your day?"

"The physical therapist came in the morning and near killed me. I thank God I have only one more session. Those people are heartless." She was in the hall, moving away.

"Doug called me at work today," Ed tried to be upbeat. "He's coming back from Aspen. Ski season is over."

"Where is he going to stay?"

"He didn't say. Probably with a friend."

"He'll be pressuring us to settle again." Her voice echoed from the bathroom.

"Probably."

A door closed and some muffled words never made it out. Ed went back to the car, picked up a six-pack of Pabst and a bottle of Jim Beam from the back seat. He placed the goods in cupboards and heard the bathroom door open and clumping of the walker. He came to help, picking up the skinny oxygen hose so Myra wouldn't get tangled.

"You didn't answer my question," she said.

"If you said something after you closed the door, I didn't hear it."

"You and your selective hearing! I asked if we had to do that mediation nonsense again."

"Doug wants to. You said absolutely not. Ms. Sanchez, the mediator, said it wouldn't go anywhere if we are so divided. She offered to mediate just for Doug and leave us out."

Myra was breathing hard as she moved closer to her recliner in front of the television, now muted. "The problem with you" —pant— "Ed, is that you" —pant— "have no backbone."

Ed stepped to the large green oxygen tank and looked at the gauge. It was less than half full. "The oxygen is on three liters a minute," he noted. "Did you turn it up?"

"No." —Gasp— "The tooth fairy did." —Pant ... pant— "Of course I did."— Gasp— "I'm not getting enough."

Her color had changed. Her lips were darker. Her fingers gripping the tubular handles were bluish. She stopped walking, pursed her lips and puffed. A couple beads of sweat sneaked out onto her forehead, bordered by half an inch of white hair under dark brown. It was a pathetically comical appearance Ed thought but never said. He had an urge to help but waited. If she could not get to and from the bathroom unassisted, she would require a higher level of temporary help. Her legs were pale. Her ankle bones were buried in edema. The tops of her feet were bulging.

"I gave you water pills this morning. Did you take them?"

"Give me a minute," she wheezed. After her efforts to breathe eased, she made the last twenty feet to her chair, smelling of urea. She positioned her rump over the target and collapsed into position. She dabbed perspiration from her face with a small towel.

"Are you taking the water pills?"

"They make me pee. It's exhausting to get to and from the bathroom."

"Maybe that's why you're having trouble breathing when you walk."

"What do you know? You're no doctor. Of course, most the ones I see are quacks, ignorant foreigners who can't hardly speak English."

"I think they are excellent for the most."

"They are so young. I can't pronounce their names and I never know who I'm going to see. It's not like it used to be. We've been overrun by the damn Indians."

Ed wanted to explain but kept silent, knowing it would only end up in an argument. Medical care was different than years earlier; that was true. Her clinic rotated internal medicine and family practitioners and few of them were American born. When he was young, his doctor did everything from broken bones to polio shots. He made house calls with a bulky leather case full of medicines. It seemed that he had all knowledge and was one of the mysterious high priests of Medicine. Ed was deeply saddened when he learned this trusted doctor from his youth had later blown his brains out.

"I saw Dr. Harrison today," he changed subjects. "He walked past my office."
"He should be in jail."
"He looked dejected."
"Couldn't happen to a nicer guy."
"I'm not so certain he did anything wrong."
"And I think you have lost your mind. What has gotten into you?"
"I'm going to check on Amy. She's been awfully quiet since coming home."

He found her in the basement, playing with some old blocks that had entertained her since she was five. The air became lighter the farther away from Myra he was. Amy smiled. They built walls and castles until they both got hungry.

CHAPTER 38

The afternoon in several rooms of Chandler Cardiovascular Clinic was filled with triumph and delicious schadenfreude. The physicians celebrated boisterously and would back-slap, chest-butt, group-hug and high-five each other in the halls. The nursing and clerical people who had worked there for over four years, gathered in corners and nooks expressing their rage, seething with resentment. The man they revered and who treated them with respect had been cheated. The celebrators had stolen the practice and by arrogance lost much of the goodwill. One conversation in the break room next to the business office involved two women.

"In the years when he ran the clinic he paid us a percentage of the profits after the physicians' income reached a certain level. That meant some huge bonuses for us. It was great."
"I wish I had worked here then."
"He made us all a part of the team, valued and rewarded. Now, we're abused and discarded without much thought."

"If Malouf yells at me one more time, I might wring her skinny neck."

"Oh, you won't be alone, honey."

"I overhear them sometimes. They make more money now that he is gone."

"We certainly don't."

"He yelled at Malouf one day. Said didn't want to go to jail for being involved with some deal."

"What deal, Andrea?"

"I don't know."

"A toast," said Monty Pierce. "To Chandler and continued success!"

Champagne glasses clinked as a dozen doctors and a couple of practice administrators savored sweet victory. A few of the doctors were Mormon and sipped sparkling apple juice.

"And a special thanks to Sarisha, who did nice work bringing this to a successful conclusion."

They all drank to that. He squeezed her arm.

She twisted away to pick up an imaginary piece of lint on the carpet. "I told you Gullimore was great."

"Where is Obi-Poku?" Pierce could not forget that the Nigerian had spoken briefly with Harrison earlier at Christianson King in a fashion that he could only interpret as friendly.

"I guess he's still working at the hospital, trying to catch up from being downtown."

Blackstone approached the pair. "Congratulations," he said. "It's a sweet moment of triumph. You did well." His gaze bounced to her chest and back to her face.

"Nice of you to say so."

"At least Nigel Sampson left with class," Blackstone said. "No suits, no anger."

"He left town," Pierce observed, "didn't break his non-compete and got all his money. He had nothing to fight about."

"True, true. He still did it with grace. He could've argued about the stock price."

"We had re-valued the stock by then," Malouf countered. "We didn't make the same mistake with Nigel that we did with Hugh. Technically, Hugh had a valid argument. It's a good thing he screwed it up and that our dog was meaner than his."

"Whatever," Stan said. "We won. He lost. Right prevailed once again. End of story."

"What's going on with your malpractice suit?" Monty asked.

"Which one?"

"You have more than one?" Blackstone said nothing.

"The one with you and Harrison," Pierce clarified.

"We had a settlement conference that died when one of the plaintiffs collapsed and broke her hip. We go to trial in July, I think. I should have been dropped from the claim but I'll be cleared. That's for sure."

"Your compassion and sensitivity are such that I'm surprised you've ever been sued."

"Thank you. Anyway, Sarisha, you earned the spacious corner office today." Blackstone then moved to another part of the room.

"How many lawsuits does he have going at the moment?" Monty asked when he was out of earshot.

"Three. Compassion and sensitivity? You've been drinking."

"That's how he sees himself. Just feeding his ego. Have you looked at his skills and outcomes?"

"They're subpar but not horrible. That said, I wouldn't let him touch me. I think he gets sued because of his personality."

"Amen to that." Pierce smiled at his own inside humor. "I assume that Chandler has been named in all of his claims."

"Every time."

"That probably increases the cost of liability insurance for everyone."

"It does."

"Well, that gives you one more thing to work on." Pierce squeezed her shoulder.

"Underway," she replied, suppressing the violent urge to smack his hand away.

Harrison's keys clattered on a table near the front door.

Beth met him as he entered the kitchen. "You're getting home a little late," she said.

"I've had a bad day." He gave her a perfunctory hug and walked to the liquor cabinet.

"You haven't answered my calls."

He poured a shot glass of tequila and gulped it down.

"Sorry. Trying to clear my head." He took another shot, then put the tequila away.

"Something bad happened at the trial?"

"The arbitration. Leo was horrible. Their attorney devoured him."

"So you lost?"

"Everything." He filled a lowball glass with ice and a slice of lime.

"They get to keep your money?"

"Yes. And I get to pay them over four hundred thousand bucks for legal costs."

"You can't be serious, Hugh. That's awful."

He poured gin two-thirds to the top and filled it the rest of the way with tonic.

"I don't have half that. They could take the house and either attach my income or take my retirement, what little I have built up since divorce." He took a large swallow.

"You oughta take it easy there, cowboy."

"Winner take all does discourage lawsuits."

"Oh, Hugh." She grasped his forearms and squeezed. Her eyes searched his face, looking concerned and he only showed bland acceptance. "Giving up and getting drunk isn't like you. Why aren't you pissed off?"

When she let go he swirled his ice cubes, looking inside the glass for an answer. "It doesn't help."

"You built the practice, took it to the top, made it a premier cardiology group. And you walk away owing them? Those guys are pure evil. It should make you livid."

"It's not much different from alimony. My ex had me removed by force from the home. Then she got the assets since the value of practice was listed on my side of ledger. Today that credit turned into a debit. Screwed twice. So, while she socializes and exercises I get to support her with six thousand dollars a month unless she marries or shacks up. This is the system."

"What about an appeal?"

"This was a binding arbitration. Appeal is not allowed." He tipped his glass and took a couple of swallows.

"How can you accept disaster so passively? That really bothers me." She left the room, wiping her cheeks.

Harrison opened the wine cabinet and peered through the small collection, finally picking a pinot noir over a chardonnay. He sat it on the counter. He put four fresh cubes in his glass, a squirt of lime, and more gin and a little tonic.

He returned to his book. He thumbed pages full of bitter humor, one that added to his despondence. The story was bleak, hopeless, pointless and highly acclaimed. He threw the paperback against a wall and looked toward the television. He rejected it as well. Returning to the kitchen, he stood, butt against the counter, icy drink cooling his fingers. There he remained numb until Beth returned.

"You're drunk. So, we shouldn't talk 'cause it will only make me mad."

"A wise choice."

"I'm sorry you lost. I can't imagine how you feel."

He emptied his glass and set it on the counter.

"I'm sure it looks bad today but tomorrow things will be a little brighter. I should stay here tonight. I worry about you."

"I'll be fine."

"Let's go out for dinner."

"I can't afford it. I'm broke."

"My treat, then. I'll drive."

"I don't feel like going out."

"You need to see there is happiness in the world."

"Every year we build a thousand libraries, each with a thousand books. Each book is filled with a hundred stories of pain. Today, I have contributed my own chapter."

"I'd like to think there are more tales of love and happiness in those libraries. So, big guy," Beth rubbed his chest, "stop wallowing. Let's go eat."

"I'd rather not."

"Please."

He walked away, to the wall where the book he hated lay splayed in despair. He picked it up and fell back to his recliner. He avoided looking in her direction but was aware she was silently crying. When she left the room he looked at the vacant space she had occupied. A yawning emptiness gaped before him. He returned to the page but the words made no sense.

He wasn't clear about how long he stayed paralyzed in disconnection. He was roused when Beth entered quietly with a nylon gym bag.

"I'm going home, Hugh."

He said nothing, waiting for more information. They looked at each other without speaking.

Beth continued. "I cleaned out my drawer."

She lifted the tote in demonstration, then plopped it on the table. Hugh put his drink down.

"I don't know if I can deal with you like this." She kissed him voraciously on the lips, hot and messy. She stroked his cheek and deep into his eyes, burning that moment into her memory forever. "Maybe it's time to cut my losses." She picked up her satchel and walked out the door, wiping her eyes.

Hugh put the book down. After the sound of her car faded some streets away, he fixed another G and T. He returned to the recliner and started to sob.

Chapter 39

A few weeks later Harrison and Damjanovich left the office of James Jenkins, a solo family lawyer in Sandy, a suburb south of Salt Lake. They had spent an hour arguing for a suspension of alimony since Harrison's financial situation had deteriorated. They got nowhere. He wouldn't be able to file a successful motion for modification until he could show his income had fallen despite his best efforts to keep it up.

That evening Harrison headed to the Apocalypse Theatre that specialized on foreign and artistic films. It was in an urban neighborhood with an array of new age shops and eateries. He hadn't been in that area for several years. Hugh had not bothered to look up what was showing. It didn't matter because he didn't want to go home to an empty life. He parked on the street half a block away, like everyone else.

There was a short line of half a dozen people and he queued up without paying much attention.

"Hugh?" A familiar face, a forty-something woman, smiled broadly at him.

"Jana," he replied. "It's been a few years."

"It's been too long."

He glanced at her left hand. "How are you?"

"I'm doing well. I'm surprised to see you here."

"We had good times here."

"I come often." She looked around. "Are you here with someone?"

"No. What about you?"

"I'm here by myself as usual." She held up a single ticket. "You look good."

"Hardly. May I join you?" He paid through the window.

"Sure. We can catch up."

He held the door open for her and smelled vanilla as she passed by. It evoked memories. Immediately inside was the candy counter. He bought two coffees, provided in ceramic cups. Inside the dimly lit auditorium, they had no trouble finding seats.

"Jana, are you still at the U in history?"

"They made me interim chair a few months ago. I've heard lots of rumors about you. What are you doing?" She put both hands around the cup to warm her fingers, just as she had years before.

"I'll be working in Arizona for a few weeks, then finding work somewhere else." He didn't want to talk about his careening career. "Department Chair! I can't imagine you like dealing with faculty problems."

"I don't. It's temporary. They offered me the position but I told them I'd only do interim until they found someone else."

"I have missed you." There was an awkward moment. "I just stopped calling back then. I'm sorry. That must have been confusing."

"I didn't think you and I would last. You know, too good to be true. I didn't know how it would end. It just faded away without…." She sighed. "Being single for the rest of my life seems like the future."

"The way I left was, I don't know, kinda vague."

"You don't need to say anything, Hugh."

"It was so soon after my marriage ended and I wanted to look around and see what kind of women were available. That sounds bad, I know."

"Uh-huh. Yeah."

"But since then I have…have come to realize…um, well, I really liked the time we spent together. Are you seeing anyone now?"

"No one steady."

The screen came to life, the music rose and conversation became difficult. Afterward he walked her to a small white Ford sedan.

"Do you want to go somewhere for a drink?" Harrison asked.

"I don't think so. This was a nice little chance meeting, one of those surprise moments. I don't want to spoil it."

"You're sure?"

She unlocked her car and opened the door. "Yeah. Last time we started too fast. We needed to develop more important things."

"Can I call you?"

They exchanged phone numbers, then hugged properly.

"Bye, Hugh," she said, then pivoted into the car and drove into the evening.

He walked past the shops dark and closed now except for a tiny coffee shop where a few theatergoers sat reveling in the company of friends. Jana had not changed much, still thin, same T-shirt, jeans, shoes, lip balm, perfume. In the years that had slid by he had learned that he did poorly in relationships. He wondered if he even wanted to try once more given the pain that invariably followed.

CHAPTER 40

Harrison zipped up his suitcase and checked his watch. His flight to Phoenix would board in two hours. He had plenty of time but was anxious so he called a taxi earlier than necessary. It was his first traveling assignment and the only cardiology work in months. He sat, tapping his foot until his phone startled him. The name Higgins Cowen appeared. He answered.

"Doctor, this is Dominici. Got a minute?"

"Yes."

"Melissa has had several exchanges with Swift. I think he's on board. We're finishing up and should be filing our complaint early next week."

"Okay. Do I need to do anything?"

"This is your last chance to bail out. Once submitted, the missile has left the silo and there's no getting it back. All kinds of grief is likely to come your way."

"I'll be out of state."

"They'll find you."

"I don't work in Salt Lake. What can they do to me?"

"Who knows. It'll be something. Keep your eyes open, Doctor."

"Press on," Harrison said. "I'm ready."

"Swift said he thought this would not take long since it's a per se violation. He's hoping for an expedited judgement in a couple of months, pretty much unheard of, really. These things usually take years. But in this case, we have more than just a smoking gun. We've got their document."

"Good to hear."

"Thank you, Doctor, for bringing this to our attention. Some of these big healthcare companies need to learn that they can't just break the law time after time."

"Right." Harrison could think of nothing to say. The issue that had not been addressed was the damage done in closing St. Lucius and the millions it cost Pacific Hospital Group. He jotted a note to remind him to call their general counsel.

"Melissa will let you know when we file. Good luck!"

They had never discussed money in all of their interactions except in vague terms. It would be a payday for Higgins Cowen and something for him.

A horn honked outside. A cab was waiting. He hurried out.

A couple hundred thousand dollars would pay off Chandler if we win this, he thought during the ride. *$10 million would come close to a break even if I lose the malpractice suit in court. Putting Blackstone and his clueless insensitivity along with me, unable to hold down a job together in front of a sympathetic jury who see the motherless impaired child every day seems like a guaranteed failure. Failure seems to be my specialty lately. I hope I don't kill anyone in Arizona.*

Chapter 41

On July 24, Pioneer Day in Utah, a big holiday, Doug Thompson was arrested with more than enough methamphetamine to meet the criteria for "intent to distribute." It was not his, of course, and he knew nothing about it. A friend of an acquaintance had given him a nylon bag to watch for the Utah holiday. Since he was out on bail, he went back to jail until his trial in a few weeks.

A few days later Ed came home from work a little after four with Amy following behind.

Myra was seated in the front room watching television, a walker next to her.

"Hart got the malpractice trial delayed to September, after Doug's trial," he said.

"How did Sarah ever get involved with that loser?"

"Careful. He's Amy's dad." Amy had already disappeared without a word. Ed made sure she was not lingering, eavesdropping. "I talked to an attorney today about Amy. He's drafting papers for us to get permanent custody."

"I can't take care of her anymore," Myra said.

"We can do this. I mean, Amy was with him in the park when he was arrested. We can't leave her with him. It's not right."

"What did we do to end up in such a mess?"

"We're in it. That's it. We should be able to restrict him to supervised visiting, no more letting Amy spend time alone with him."

"That gives us no freedom."

"As if we had any."

Ed felt trapped by both of the women in his life so his words came out a bit harsh. Myra took no notice.

"How's the hip?" he asked.

"Killing me."

"Have you been up like the doctor said?"

"Of course." Ed knew this was a lie. Facade was ingrained in their relationship.

"Let me help you up and walk outside on sidewalk. It's not too hot right now. Then I'll cook dinner."

"I remember taking walks with you and Sarah when she was about Amy's age," Myra said. "I was a lot smaller then."

"It was before you had the thyroid problem." Ed noticed a softening in her attitude.

"And before Sarah passed. I've put on so much fat."

"It's been hard."

"I hope I was a good mother."

"She thought so."

"If I had been better maybe she would've chosen a decent husband."

"She didn't marry him because he was a good catch."

"She should have had an abortion."

"Then we wouldn't have Amy."

"Exactly."

She's the one bright spot in my life, he thought. *She's the only thing that gives any meaning to anything I do.* "Let's take a walk, Myra."

"I've been up enough," she said.

"Doctor said to get outside when you can."

"I know what the idiot said."

She turned the volume up on the TV set. Ed sighed and walked to the kitchen. He pulled out a beer.

She called out, "Bring me a couple of Percodan, Ed."

Since the trial had been postponed, Harrison was trying to find some temporary work in

August. Manhattan Kansas needed an inventional cardiologist. Hugh had applied through

Walthrop Locum Tenens and was on the phone with Nigel, a recruiter.

"Why do they need a temp cardiologist?"

"One lost his license after sleeping with a patient, an associate professor of dairy science at Kansas State," Nigel said, amused. "A woman. That's off the record."

"That's funny?"

"We've made so many jokes about that in the office."

"Milk-producing glands?"

"Exactly."

"When could I start? I'm now available in August."

"The hospital has a problem with you. We're trying to work through that."

"A problem?" Harrison asked.

"Auspicious Health owns the hospital. Apparently someone at the top has an issue."

"I see."

"Is there something I should know about?" Nigel asked. "What's up?"

"I got sideways with one of their hospitals in Salt Lake. Nothing medical. I'm kind of a witness against them for some shady financial doings."

"You're the only clean candidate we've presented and it looks like they prefer someone else, one with some drug history. I hope we can put you there but it's not looking good."

"What else have you got besides Kansas?"

"North Dakota and Oregon but you're not licensed in either state. Dakota doesn't take long but Oregon is at least six months. So, right now I've got nothing else interventional. We can get you something in general cardiology, non-invasive that is, at a couple of VA hospitals."

"I can't stand non-invasive," Harrison said. "I'll need to think about that."

"Okay if we start a license application in Oregon and North Dakota?"

"Get it started." He hung up, discouraged. This was the second time he had been blocked from working by Auspicious. He was getting desperate. He had paid June half of her alimony for July and a letter from her attorney sat unopened on his kitchen table. The next extortion was due in three days and if he paid what she demanded he would have less than a thousand dollars for the rest of the month. It was going to get ugly. He was desperate for work. He dialed the number for Loco Locums, a little start up in Dallas, hoping to find something.

The malpractice trial was about to start. Zone and Hayes wanted to be present for the jury selection. Hayes' task was to look into each prospective juror to see if they had a grievance, an unpaid hospital bill or, worse, if they had been sent to collections.

"You saw Myra Szabo on the outlier report," Zone asked as they were half-way downtown.

"She's been on the list for almost a week."

Patients whose costs had exceeded their payments were listed there and got special attention to grease the skids out of the hospital. Myra was hospitalized again, this time in intensive care at OCHA, her lungs pumped by the bellows of a mechanical ventilator. She had failed at least four attempts to wean her off the support. In the ten days she had been ill she had seldom been fully awake. She almost certainly had no idea the trial was finally getting underway.

"Isn't this ironic," Zone said. "She's suing us for millions. Yet, here she is, costing us more than Medicare pays."

"I don't think her intent was to get so sick she would spend weeks in the ICU."

"Karma then?"

"Whose? Hers for being annoying or ours for the death of her daughter?"

He looked at Hayes confused.

"Never mind. That was a little deep for a jock," she said. "Are you saying we could lose this?" he asked.

"The malpractice? The fight is between Blackstone and Harrison. I don't see why we should lose."

"We have the deep pockets."

"Our guy, Parr, just needs to point out at every turn that we have high-quality data, that we have high standards for credentialing and that we cannot referee all of the petty disagreements between egocentric narcissists. We'll be fine."

"I hope so."

Inside the courthouse they were soon joined by a pair of Auspicious Healthcare executives from Nashville who took part in the early morning protracted excoriation. They sat together two rows back. Seated in front of them at the plaintiff's table were Dennis Hart and Ed Szabo. Hart wore a dark blue suit and a tie that featured red. His full head of salt-and-pepper hair and his reading glasses gave an unmistakable impression of legal warrior, staunch defender of the weak and abused. Ed wore an old brown suit.

Five people crowded behind the defendant's table. Stan Henriod on the aisle looked rumpled and well fed, brushing Krispy Kreme from his pants. Matthew Parr sat on the outside, average and unnoticeable, a middle-aged Salt Lake clone, father of four lovely girls who lived in a yuppie ghetto in Murray. He was the attorney for OCHA. Jessop was tall and striking in comparison, the image of professional. Black suit, blue blouse, and a crucifix. To her right was Dr. Blackstone, who appeared in a new charcoal suit instead of his usual mismatch. Harrison sat to Jessop left in the same pinstripe he always wore. Pope sat immediately behind them. Over twenty people, mostly from the jury pool, were scattered in seats, quiet and intimidated by the circumstances and most wishing to be almost anywhere else.

The judge entered with the usual fanfare, all rising and being seated. She was a squat woman, oval face, large nose, black hair graying at the temples, who spoke exquisite American English with shades of New England aristocracy. She was married to a physician, an elite radiation oncologist at the University and a Boston Brahmin. She, Rosa Bradford, was the best Judge Hart could have wanted based on her track record in personal injury cases.

Bradford requested attorneys from each side of the room to approach the bench. "Have your clients settled this morning?"

"No, Your Honor," Hart answered.

"Did you try?"

She scowled at the lack of any answer. "Few if any of these cases should ever make it to trial. I see four plaintiffs listed and but one at your table, Counselor. Do they not take this process seriously?"

"Indeed they do, Your Honor. One is a minor and in school. Her father is technically not a plaintiff. He is in jail, arrested on an unrelated matter. Mrs. Szabo is hospitalized in intensive care."

"I'm sorry to hear that. You are not filing for another continuance then?"

"No, Your Honor."

"Are all of your plaintiffs agreeable to starting today?"

"Yes, Your Honor. They are all very anxious to bring this matter to a conclusion."

"I take it then there are no last-minute motions. Let's get this jury selected."

The questions began. Decisions were easy for Hart. On the other side of the room, however, several attorneys had to confer, disagree, discuss and debate before they could accept or reject each juror. After the gamut had been run and the selections made, they dispersed for lunch, grateful it took only half a day.

Outside under an overcast sky, Harrison checked his voicemail. His phone had vibrated with a couple of calls he could not answer during the morning session. One was a message from Lisa Jacobs of Higgins Cowen. She needed to give him an update. He stored it rather than calling.

The other news was terse. "This is Leo. I heard from James Jenkins. He says you missed paying alimony. He's threatening to ask the court to hold you in contempt. I don't do family law, Hugh. I'll have someone call you that does. But, call me. We should talk."

Hugh tried to eat a sandwich he brought with him while sitting in his car in the underground lot. He was tired of lawyers and suffocated by financial futility. He had a high-income profession, but money was sucked away in every direction. He put the key in the ignition and considered driving far away. Belize seemed like a good destination. He stared through the windshield at a cement wall for a while in depression. He put the key in his pocket and ambled unwillingly back to the battle with a new appreciation of why apparently successful people sometimes off themselves.

With the jury impaneled court convened at two o'clock. Amy was there. Her features were a constant reminder to the jury that her heightened needs must be met. A drawing book, with colored pencils and crayons occupied the outside part of the table, right in front of the jury box. Hart adjusted his cuffs and tie then began.

"On April 13, 2004, Sarah Thompson, the mother of Amy, seated here at the table with her grandfather, Ed, became ill with a stomachache. Twelve days later, she was dead and Amy was motherless. Ed and Myra Szabo, Sarah's parents, lost their only daughter. The death of a young mother is always tragic. It's a sad fact of life that hundreds of young people die in this country every day. There's little we can do to change that. Nothing we accomplish in court this week will bring Sarah back. However, if you come to believe as I do, that the two doctors seated across the room and the hospital where they practiced failed to treat her with requisite skill and competence, you can help right a wrong. Having snuffed out this young mother's life, as recompense they should support her daughter Amy. This is a simple concept, one that has been used for thousands of years. We ask not an eye for an eye or a life for a life but the Biblical rule that restitution is threefold.

"We have an expectation of good care when we go to any hospital. If we need a specialist, we expect the highest level of expertise. Sarah saw an internal medicine physician when she was admitted to Olympus Center of Healing Arts, a hospital we all call OCHA. We have not included either of the two internists who were involved in her care in this claim because after careful review we found they performed well. Cardiologists are specialists in heart disease that get years of additional training after training in internal medicine. The two physicians seated at the defendant's table fit into that category," he spoke as he pointed. "Some cardiologists specialize in heart failure. No such sub-specialist was involved in the care of Sarah until it was too late.

"The defense will argue, of course, that Sarah had a disease that was fatal, that even in the best of hands she would have died. This is simply untrue. Her illness had a cure that has been effective for years. She was denied access to the cure by the two doctors on trial and by the hospital where she was treated for ten days. She deteriorated daily as Dr. Harrison watched and persisted in providing what our experts will testify was unproven and harmful therapy. When Dr. Blackstone took over her case, she continued to fail. When she was finally at death's door, he delayed in sending her to the heart failure center at Wasatch Hospital, where it was too late to save her.

"The unproven treatments rendered at OCHA and delays in proper referral are the reasons we seek damages. There is every reason to believe that Sarah Thompson would be alive, gainfully employed and taking care of her daughter today, had she been appropriately treated. Failing to exercise scientific and compassionate care, these two doctors deprived Sarah of the chance to live. We believe that the financial burden of caring for Amy, the young daughter who has Down syndrome and will need lifelong support, should fall upon those physicians who failed to meet the minimum standards of care.

"You will hear testimony of several expert witnesses, highly qualified heart failure specialists, that will dissect the actions of these two men and find them wanting. The single expert testifying for the defense will have an impossible task as you will readily see. Remember this one overriding fact as you deliberate. Sarah would probably be alive today if she had been referred earlier to the level of care she required. The days of delay cost her life. The financial support Sarah would have provided now, if justice is to be served, should fall on those who erred, whose malpractice resulted in this tragedy. Simple justice is all we seek."

Hart walked back to his table, pausing above Amy as she was clumsily coloring.

Jessop stood to deliver the opening statement of all defendants. "Mr. Hart would have you believe that these caregivers are heartless, that they went through more than a decade of education and training, of privation and sacrifice just to carelessly watch people die. There is no rationale to support Mr. Hart's contentions about any of the defendants.

"The death of Sarah Thompson pains us all. When we see the life of a mother in her prime snuffed out, we think, 'Perhaps, but for the grace of God, there go I.' The doctors and hospital expended every reasonable effort to save Sarah's life. As you will soon learn in detail she had a one hundred percent fatal disease. Hers was a rare kind of myocarditis. You will learn that almost all people with myocarditis get better on their own. No one has found a medical treatment proven to be of benefit in any form of myocarditis, including the invariably fatal variant that killed Sarah.

"The two cardiologists seated before you are brilliant and well educated. Like all of us, they are not perfect. If we required perfection in physicians, we would have none. Would Sarah be alive today if she had received a heart transplant? Perhaps. This is Mr. Hart's claim and the ploy to extract tens of millions of dollars from the healthcare industry that keeps you all alive and well. When a large amount of money is involved, one must be cautious about the arguments and statements used to support the claim. Mr. Hart has asked for thirty million dollars.

"The defense of the accusations is not a disregard for Sarah's life. It is sometimes in our nature to blame someone for an untimely death. Mr. Hart wants to lay it at the feet of the doctors and hospital. OCHA has excellent objective public data supporting it as an excellent center for cardiac patients. Mr. Hart will undoubtedly provide inaccurate portrayals of both physicians and a host of overly optimistic what-ifs for you to consider. All I ask is for you to look at the facts and make a decision based on them, not out of pity for this cute little girl or righteous indignation or for some other emotion. Facts, not opinions. That's all I ask, all that the community requires, and all the judge expects. Justice is blind. Facts, facts, facts. Look at them carefully and you will reach a conclusion, I predict, that neither these physicians nor Olympus Hospital is to blame for the death of Sarah Thompson. Thank you."

CHAPTER 41

Ed Szabo was called first. He walked easily to the stand in his brown suit, threadbare at the elbows, tattered hems, and lapels too wide. He spent an hour in the box answering questions stoically without expression. Following a recess, Henriod cross-examined him. Jessop took notes and formulated questions.

As Henriod was concluding, Harrison looked over her notes and whispered to her. "Do you really need to ask him any questions?"

"I have a couple of things I'd like to clarify."

"He's a grieving parent who's looking awfully sympathetic. I don't want the jury to think—"

"I know what I'm doing."

Harrison backed off. She crossed off several questions. Henriod sat.

"Any questions, Ms. Jessop?"

She stood, still shuffling her papers. "Very briefly, Your Honor. Mr. Szabo, did you or your wife to your knowledge ever make an attempt to speak with Dr. Harrison while Sarah was alive?"

"We never met him."

"Did you try?"

"He never came around when we visited."

"What time did you visit?"

"In the evenings."

"May we assume from your answers that other than visiting Sarah in the evening that you did not make a specific attempt to be present when the physician made rounds?"

"Not that I recall."

"I'm sorry, Mr. Szabo. I need an answer that is clear. Yes or no, did you try to speak with

Dr. Harrison?"

He paused.

"Please, Mr. Szabo," the judge directed.

"She said the doctor wouldn't let her go home. She wanted to get back to work. Honestly, she didn't seem very sick to us so we didn't speak with Dr. Harrison."

"So you didn't really try?" Jessop prodded.

"I came to see Sarah after work. I didn't take time off to hang around waiting for him to show up."

"You said she didn't seem very sick." Jessop paused and threw a glance at Pope. "Interesting. She looked normal to you?"

"She was a little pale but she looked that way every April when she worked a hundred hours a week."

"When did she start to look sick?"

"After she was in the ICU on Saturday."

"Not when Dr. Harrison was taking care of her."

Henriod scooted his chair noisily back and sat on edge, ready to leap to his feet. Pope cleared his throat.

"Right."

"Thank you. I am sorry for your loss, sir." Monica returned to the defense table. "That's all for me, Your Honor."

Henriod was on his feet before she reached the table.

"Does it make sense to you, Mr. Szabo, that she would be moved to the ICU because she was getting worse?"

"That would make sense if that's what happened. But it didn't happen that way."

Henriod seemed taken aback. Pope coughed and Henriod turned around. Pope made a subtle gesture. "One moment, Your Honor," Henriod said. He approached Pope and they whispered so low that Hugh could not hear.

Jessop whispered to Harrison. "They didn't like the door I opened."

Henriod wheeled around on his heel and resumed. "Dr. Blackstone gave Sarah as well as you and your wife detailed information about her condition on Saturday, correct?"

"He did."

"Did he tell you she had a serious, life-threatening condition?"

"Yes."

"And that she needed intensive care."

"He moved her there to change her treatment."

"That seems reasonable since she was deteriorating."

"Objection!" Hart stood. "Mr. Henriod is testifying." Hart caught himself. "Actually, I withdraw my objection."

"Regardless, the jury should ignore that last remark by Mr. Henriod."

"I have no more questions at this time for Mr. Szabo," Henriod said.

Matt Parr stood and began asking more questions about Ed's experience with the hospital and the personnel.

"What in the heck was that?" Henriod whispered during Parr's session.

"It's called affirmative defense. You should try it sometime."

"Ah, jeez," he said.

Ed testified that the Saturday afternoon ICU nurse was irritated, brusque. She strained to be nice to the family but seemed overwhelmed with the enormity of the task as his daughter slipped away from cogent to comatose.

"So, all in all, at the end of her shift, were you unhappy with the ICU nurse?"

"She either had inadequate support or was put in a no-win situation. I have nothing against her."

This is not an angry man, Hugh thought. *And Parr is a moron, working for the plaintiffs.*

That evening, hoping to have company, Hugh made spaghetti sauce from whole tomatoes, fresh basil, oregano, onions, peppers, garlic and some red wine. He rolled meatballs, cut fresh bread and boiled linguini. A pair of tall candles flickered over a pale yellow tablecloth, Verdi slid quietly out of small speakers, the chandelier in the dining nook was dimmed. The little dining space was a stark contrast to the rest of the apartment. Dozens of cardboard boxes of various sizes were stacked along the walls.

This was one meal he loved to cook, one full of pleasant memories. He had called Jana after court and left her a message. It looked like he would enjoy this one alone. His phone jangled and his spirits went up until he saw it was a San Francisco area code for the second time that day.

"Harrison."

"Dr. Harrison, this is Lisa Jacobs with Higgins Cowen."

"Hi. What's up?"

"Sorry to call so late. Do you have a minute?"

"Sure. Go ahead." He wondered what the whistleblower firm had to say.

"This might take a bit longer."

"I'm in the middle of cooking dinner. Have you eaten?"

"No. I was going to fly back but it went late and there's more tomorrow."

"How about we talk over dinner?"

Silence.

"I'm not hitting on you. When I'm out of town I don't enjoy eating out alone."

"I was just thinking it over."

"I just made spaghetti and my apartment is not far from downtown. It's a mess. I just moved in. Or I could meet you at a restaurant. Either way it won't take much of your time."

Hugh didn't want to waste his shrinking funds on eating out.

"Oh. Okay. Where do you live?"

He gave her his address and simple directions. "It'll take five minutes to get here."

Six minutes later, Hugh brought her in from the street and up to his new place. "Sorry for the mess."

"It smells really good." She smiled.

"Wine?" Hugh asked, holding up a bottle of red.

"Please," she answered.

They filled plates and sat. She looked tired, he thought.

"A question or two came up in the course of the conversation this afternoon," she said.

Have you experienced any retribution from the hospital recently?"

"I lost a couple of assignments at Auspicious hospitals. Someone from corporate gives negative information to the hospitals and the assignment goes to someone else."

"Can you find out who?"

"No. I've tried. Hospitals where the company tries to send me first have to grant me hospital privileges. Part of that process involves talking anonymously to other docs and hospitals where I have worked to see if I am a problem."

"What about the locum company?" Lisa asked. "Can they tell you anything?"

"They're in the dark, so they say."

"No specifics?"

"The open malpractice case gets mentioned. The trial just started."

There was a lull in conversation as they ate, a comfortable silence.

"So, this has affected your income," Lisa stated.

"I'm living on what I got when I sold my house, whatever doesn't go to my ex. A few long weekends of work don't provide much."

"How's your case going?"

"Hard to say. It's only been one day."

"How much are they going after?"

"Thirty million."

Her eyes went large.

"Just ten from me," he said.

"Just ten," she said. "No wonder hospitals are nervous about hiring you, even as a temp.

Why so much?"

"Unexpected death of a young single mother with a special needs child."

She whistled. "Whoa. So…." She searched for the right words.

"Did I screw up? I didn't think so but in retrospect I probably should have transferred her instead of letting my boneheaded partner kill her."

"So, he did something wrong?"

"She crashed when he changed her meds. But what got this whole lawsuit started was when he brazenly criticized my care to the family. Then she died."

"Did you try to settle?"

"It fell apart. So, why did you call?"

"Oh, yeah," she said, savored a bite, and washed down with the wine. "I sat in on a couple of the conversations Swift had with Auspicious." She tapped her temple.

"Their attorney was pretty convincing that the agreement was clean. He's wrong, of course, but he makes sincere sounding arguments. He was not going to settle, that was pretty clear. And Gullimore, the attorney for your old group, was adamant, bordering on angry. He had nothing but vitriol for you and threatened to sue you for slander."

"All I need right now is another legal complication."

"You've made no public statements, so he was just blowing smoke. But you should know what's in the wind."

"I appreciate that."

"Tomorrow we meet with the judge. He'll find out there's no plea, no settlement and no promising negotiation. Then he'll throw out the motion to dismiss then we'll wade into the weeds about the consent decree and the contract that you provided. They want that thrown out, of course, because they claim it wasn't obtained legally. That's our biggest risk. If that's gone, the case won't hold up."

"Do you think he'll allow it?"

"He should. It depends on how your agreement is interpreted, their narrow way or what it literally says." She paused to eat. A comfortable quiet buoyed the room. "This is delicious. You made this?"

"I had a good teacher. What are the chances he'll allow it?"

"One hundred percent if he understands English and ten percent if he's buddies with someone on their side, a former partner, a paramour, a member of his club or fraternity or church. I don't know the down and dirty on judges in Utah."

"That's it? A crap shoot?"

"We get good judges and we get some others." She scooted away from the table and stepped to her small briefcase. She pulled out a manila folder, flipped through a few dozen pages and pulled out a laser printed clean white sheet. She came back to the table, sat and sipped her wine.

Hugh watched and waited without a word.

"He's Presbyterian, not a Mormon," she read. "He was a Pi Kap, as was one of Gullimore's senior partner. They go to the same church on South Temple."

"You do research on judges?"

"Out of necessity."

"Oh, man." He put his face in his hands.

"It's too soon to worry, Dr. Harrison. Let's see the direction this takes. So, now give me specifics. What hospitals did not offer you work?"

CHAPTER 42

Dr. William F. Grainger, a large man with a short, professorial beard, blue blazer and gray slacks, launched a blistering, methodical and comprehensive assault on Harrison that lasted ninety minutes. He displayed an occasional hint of Minnesota accent in his otherwise plain English. Hart's junior associate, Brett Rasmussen, guided the barrage with slanted questions as Hart had remained at the desk. Ramussen's medical background made him facile with technical jargon.

Jessop didn't wait for him to sit before she began hurling her cross-examination questions. "Dr. Grainger, you currently work at the heart failure clinic at Hemerton Memorial in Massachusetts, correct?"

His chin went up. "Indeed I do."

"In what capacity?"

"I hold the Pettigrew Chair. I run the heart failure group."

"Is Hemerton considered a prestigious hospital?"

"We have an excellent reputation and compare well with the Boston facilities."

"I imagine competition for your position was fierce, was it not?"

"There were a large number of highly qualified applicants."

"So, you might say you were the best of the best?" The jury saw a faint smirk on her face and perked up.

"My training and publications are impeccable."

"How well do your heart failure patients fare?"

He looked at the jury. "We have a great program."

"Your Honor," Monica said as she hoisted several sheets of paper, "I would like to introduce this report into evidence. It deals with the credibility and quality of this expert."

"What is it?"

"A report from ReportCardMedical. It shows patient mortality rates at all hospitals in Massachusetts."

"Objection," Hart stood. "Relevance."

"Overruled," Judge Bradford stated. "It's impeachment evidence."

One copy went to Hart and another received a sticker from the court reporter, logged and entered into evidence as Jessop waited.

"Thank you, Your Honor. Now, Dr. Grainger, please look at this report. Where is Hemerton Memorial listed?"

It took him a while to read through the names. "It is at the bottom," he replied.

"The list is ranked from best to worst with the A facilities at the top and E rankings at the bottom," Jessop said. "Are you familiar with ReportCard, Doctor?"

"No," he stated, waving his hand dismissively. "And our care does not deserve an E. Our data are more reliable and do not agree with this junk."

"Please look at North Shore Medical Center near the top of the list. What is their predicted and actual mortality?"

Reluctantly he reopened the sheaf. "Predicted mortality was 3 percent. Actual mortality was almost 2 percent."

"1.7 percent, actually. Now look at your program at the very bottom. Tell the jury what those same statistics are for your place."

"Like I said, our own numbers are more accurate and reflect a high quality on a par with Mass General."

"Please answer the question," Jessop pressed.

He squirmed and adjusted his tortoise reading glasses. "This is not accurate information."

Jessop appealed to the judge with a gesture. She spoke. "Doctor, please answer." "Predicted mortality was 5 percent. Actual mortality was 13 percent."

"So, by these numbers, Hemerton heart failure patients are seven times more likely to die than patients at North Shore, correct?"

"As I said, I don't believe this data."

He displayed confidence and challenge as he lowered at Monica. She stepped closer.

"Whether you believe it or not does not matter. It is the published outcome information derived from several objective databases. Is death is an equivocal endpoint?"

"Of course not."

"It indicates your patients are far more likely to die than those at the best hospitals. Your program is ranked dead last in the state as you read from that report. Now, Doctor, you criticized Dr. Harrison for his use of carvedilol, did you not?"

"I did."

"What specific study shows it to be harmful in myocarditis?"

"It has never been studied in myocarditis."

"Never?" Monica returned to the table and Hugh slid another sheet to her. She held it up and approached the judge. "Your Honor, I would like to introduce this paper, an abstract of a study of carvedilol in acute myocarditis presented in 2003." After it had been logged, she placed it before the witness. "I'll give you a minute to look over the study that you just testified under oath did not exist."

She stood next to the jury box and waited, looking frequently at her watch. When his eyes came up, she spoke.

"Is that a study of carvedilol in patients with myocarditis?"

"It is a very small trial, twenty-four patients."

"Doctor, I grow tired of asking questions that you fail to answer. Please."

He looked for help from Hart, who simply raised his eyebrows. "Yes, it is such a trial." "Based on your expert testimony, it appears you are not familiar with this trial, correct?" "It was too small for me to consider it."

"I find that strange from an academic of high standing who is called to testify on that precise subject. Doctor, who did better in this trial, patients that received the same medication given to Sarah Thompson or those given placebo?"

"The findings are far from conclusive."

Jessop struck the dais in front of the witness. "Just answer the question." The resounding slap and raised voice made his eyes wide. He turned toward the judge, who glared down at him.

"Doctor, we have no time for games."

Grainger looked at the paper. "Those that received carvedilol had a twenty-five percent mortality rate while half the placebo group died. The difference was not significant."

She turned to face the jurors. "I think most of the jury would prefer to be in the group with a higher survival rate, wouldn't you?"

"I would need to look deeper into the study. This trial was done in Europe."

"In light of this study, do you still maintain that Dr. Harrison contributed to the death of Sarah Thompson by using the drug in question? Yes or no, Doctor?"

"This is only an abstract and the study is too small to be conclusive. No Americans use carvedilol in this situation as it is outside the guidelines and not—"

"Yes or no?" Jessop stood next to the jury.

"Approach?" Dennis Hart was standing.

"After he answers the question," the judge said.

"It's not clear."

"Yes or no?" Jessop asked again, clearly out of patience. "Is there any trial in medical literature that supports your opinion that the use of this beta blocker drug contributed to the death of Sarah Thompson?"

William Grainger's voice was paralyzed. His lips were moving fishlike. "Not to my knowledge."

Judge Bradford motioned to Hart, who waved her off and sat down, no longer wanting a side bar.

Monica reviewed her notes on the table and came back to the witness, who was mopping his head and eyes with a white handkerchief. She turned her back to the cardiologist and faced the jury. "I am almost finished, Dr. Grainger. One small issue to clarify. In your written report and again on the stand this morning you criticized Dr. Harrison for not using the cardiac stimulant drug dobutamine, did you not?"

"Yes."

"Nice, concise answer, Doctor. Thank you."

He bristled at her condescension. She still faced the jury, watching their faces.

"In a heart failure patient such as Mrs. Thompson, please explain to us when this drug most helpful?"

"It is used when the cardiac output is low enough to cause poor urine output or other evidence of shock. We give intermittent infusions to improve symptoms of heart failure."

"What symptoms did Mrs. Thompson have that would have been helped with dobutamine during the period my client, Dr. Harrison managed her condition?"

"Shortness of breath."

"Where in the medical record did it report shortness of breath?"

"I can't remember."

Monica went to the table that held the labeled evidence, hoisted the binder that held the records from OCHA and carried it to Grainger. "Would you care to find such a statement?"

"It may take a while," he said as he took the loose-leaf and opened it up.

"It will take a very long time," Jessop said. "There was one such complaint while my client was in town. It is found on page one hundred eighty-one, the seventh day of her hospitalization. It is a nurse's note. Could you find it and read it for us?"

It took a while for him to find the page. "Patient mild S.O.B. post amb in room."

"Please tell us what that means."

"She had mild shortness of breath after walking in her room."

"After seven days of minimal activity and mostly bedrest, is that uncommon in a patient without heart failure?"

"I suppose not," he admitted.

Monica paced thoughtfully between the witness and jury boxes, fingering her gold cross, looking between the ceiling and the floor. "So, Doctor, if she did not have much shortness of breath, did she have poor urinary output?"

"I don't recall that she did."

"So, if she had mild and infrequent difficulty breathing and good kidney function, what would be the benefit from dobutamine while Dr. Harrison took care of Mrs. Thompson?"

"It would have improved her cardiac function."

"This drug has been used and studied for decades, is that a fair statement?"

"Yes."

"How many of these studies have shown benefit in curing or improving myocarditis?"

"None." He answered cautiously.

"Does this drug improve the mortality rate in heart failure in general?"

"No."

"Is it not true that in most trials an increased mortality rate is found?"

"That is true."

"How would Mrs. Thompson have benefitted from the drug you recommended when her symptoms were mild, her renal function normal and the medicine increases the probability of death?"

He sat blinking. "It's how these patients are best treated."

"Perhaps, Doctor, could your misuse of dobutamine explain why the death rate of your patients is so abysmally high?"

He gaped.

"You don't need to answer. No further questions."

Henriod came forward to cross-examine but had few questions. Parr asked enough questions to bring the clock close to noon. Judge Bradford called for lunch recess.

Chapter 43

Ed Szabo had been watching Harrison and Blackstone off and on all morning. Blackstone scowled at times at his former partner. He could not sit still and continually picked at his fingernails or twisted cloth or paper in tension. He pulled cards from his coat pocket and read them, lips moving. He closed his eyes in deep concentration for brief moments. In short he appeared as a man in turmoil. As Harrison walked out of the room without expression, Blackstone's eyes followed him, the look on his face angry. After two days of observing the dynamic between the two men, the damning statement from Blackstone three years earlier, the singular phrase that initiated this entire process, assumed a different meaning to Ed.

"Bring the little girl with you to my office for lunch," Hart told Ed.

Her name is Amy, Ed thought. Hart had requested that Amy appear at the morning session. She had been well behaved as she normally was. Ed wanted to get her back to school. Amy had been seen more than enough for the day.

He could not decide if there was enough time to get her back, however. He put her coloring book and crayons in her pink Spice Girls backpack and walked out in search of restrooms.

"School ... now?" Her speech was not improving and Ed felt guilty he could not work with her enough.

"Mr. Hart wants to give us lunch, Amy."

"Car?"

"There's not enough time to get you there and come back." There was also the uncertainty of when he would get away from the trial in the afternoon. He wanted to promise her she could go to school tomorrow but he said nothing.

Blackstone overheard the conversation as he and Stacey, his wife, walked by. He leaned to his wife's ear, saying, "Her father is in jail for drugs, a real loser. God only knows what her mother did to bring this upon her daughter. The sins of the parents have been visited upon the head of their daughter."

"The fathers have eaten a sour grape and the children's teeth are set on edge."

"Proverbs, right?"

"No. Jeremiah 31 and in Ezekiel as well," she corrected.

"Oh, that's right. At any rate, we are truly blessed with a beautiful child."

"By the grace of God."

"We obey laws of nature, man and God and are blessed because of it and yet we say it is by grace that we are well off. Maybe it's grace plus talent and work."

"It is by grace. We're one accident, one disease away from poverty."

"I know. It's by grace that I have talent and a great practice.

"As far as your practice is concerned, you did not start it, neither do you run it. Others have done much of the work that benefits us. You opposed building the cath lab but it has almost doubled our income, hasn't it?"

"After we made a deal with OCHA, the money came rolling in. I supported that."

"Dr. Harrison never saw any of that money, did he?"

"Not a penny. In fact, he's paying us." He smiled.

"One man reaps what another sows."

"Harrison is kind of an antichrist, an atheist."

"We are charitable, dear. Full of love for all. Love thine enemy."

"I fall far short of that."

Ed had overheard the first part of Blackstone's declaration but nothing showed on his face. He and Amy found the ladies restroom but at the door Amy held fast to his arm.

"What's wrong, honey?"

"Afraid."

Harrison and Jessop passed by at that moment. Jessop stopped.

"Hi, Ed," Harrison said. "Need some help?"

"She's a little nervous but we'll be fine," he replied.

"I'll take her in there, if that would help," Jessop said.

"It's okay," Ed said. "She'll be fine."

Amy leaned up against her grandfather.

"Can I help?" Jessop asked, bent over, cross dangling in midair. Her white teeth glistened, as did her lips.

Lacey's green and brown eyes met Ed's then returned to Amy, who had loosened her grip.

My God, she is beautiful, he thought.

"Amy, you can go with this lady, if you want. She'll watch out for you."

"Of course I will," Lacey said and extended her hand.

Amy hesitated but relented, taking her fingers in a small grip. She handed her backpack to Ed, then walked away, looking between him and Monica.

"Cute kid," Hugh said.

"She needs her mother," he responded icily.

"You're a good man to take over in an impossible situation. She really loves you."

"You gotta do what you gotta do. It's not what I had planned."

"I hear you. Her dad seems to be troubled."

"You think?" Ed could have been friendly. It was enough to be civil. His feelings about

Dr. Harrison were conflicted.

"How's your wife?"

"I really don't want to talk about that," he answered. A long, uncomfortable pause followed, with shifting of feet and changing postures. Ed sighed.

"She has been in the ICU for eleven days now. They can't seem to get her off the ventilator."

"Sorry to hear that."

"It's been rough on her."

"People who spend that much time in the ICU always need a lot of physical rehabilitation afterward. I guess they've told you that."

"I won't be able to take care of her at home, so they say. I've been looking at nursing homes and rehabilitation."

"That plus this plus sole parent of Amy—that's gotta be rough."

Another awkward pause preceded Amy emerging, followed by Monica.

"Would you mind watching her while I visit the washroom?" Ed asked her.

"Not at all," Jessop answered.

Harrison's phone vibrated as Ed left. "Hi, Jana. What's up?"

"I'm in the courthouse, looking for you. Where are you?"

"Fourth floor. I thought you had meetings and work."

"I got away for lunch. I'll be up in a minute." True to her word she arrived quickly. "Parking here is a disaster. Hi, Hugh." She pecked him on the lips.

He introduced her to Jessop and Amy.

Jana crouched. "Aren't you supposed to be in school, young lady?"

"Yes."

"Thanks," Ed said, a hint of smile stretching his wrinkles. "Let's go to lunch, Amy."

"School," she pouted as she planted her feet.

"I don't have time, Amy. Please, let's go." He held his hand down so she would hold it and walk together.

She did not move.

"Where is her school?" Jessop asked.

"Winkler. Please, Amy. Mr. Hart is expecting us."

"That's not too far from where I work," Jana said. "I'll be going there in a few minutes, after we eat." She held up a fragrant Quiznos sack.

"I think I'll drive her there myself," Ed said. "Thanks for the offer."

"I'm going that direction anyway," Jana argued. "Save some gas and your time."

"I couldn't do that. She is my responsibility."

"I'm happy to take her. Honestly, it's no trouble."

"Let's go to my car, Amy."

As her hand came up to his, her pout dissolved and off they went, Ed hurrying as much as he could to try to make it back before the trial recommenced in the afternoon. He was conflicted about Harrison. He had been very nice, maybe to curry favor or maybe he was just a nice person. It was impossible to determine.

Dr. Paulette Neville, a short, bespectacled, plain-looking woman, had watched the morning session, particularly the cross-examination of the expert witness. She was the second expert, from the Cleveland Clinic where she had worked for eleven years. This followed a fifteen-year appointment at the University of Louisville, where she had been involved in the artificial heart program. The list of her publications in heart failure was long even when it excluded quite a number of requested articles for the "throw away" medical journals. She had testified as an expert witness over a dozen times in the last few years. She had never seen another expert so thoroughly embarrassed as Grainger.

"Are you joining us for lunch?" Hart asked her.

"I need some time alone to go over my notes and report. That was a brutal beating."

"I didn't see that coming," Grainger said, shaking his head.

"I was also unaware of that small study the defense attorney produced. That's a killer. Could I get a copy of it?"

"It's not about giant cell myocarditis," Grainger said. "I should have mentioned that."

Hart hefted his briefcase and pawed through papers and produced it. "Let's go to my office. I'll have my secretary order some sandwiches. You have to make a copy and a secluded corner to hunker down."

Paulette read as they walked. As she did so, she realized she had to either revise her testimony or lose professional credibility. She was being paid to testify to something that was challenged by the latest data and this made her squirm. Six hundred fifty dollars an hour was twice what she made at the clinic. These high-paying gigs provided nice gifts for her three grandchildren in Connecticut. A bad performance would jeopardize that. For the next hour she chewed on conflicts and conundrums.

After dropping Amy at the school, Ed stopped in at his home to grab a quick sandwich he could eat as he drove back. There was a light blinking on his answering machine. He tapped the playback button on his way to the refrigerator.

"Mr. Szabo, this is Bull, the nurse taking care of your wife. It's nine-thirty A.M. on Tuesday. Please call me as soon as you get this message."

"Damn it," he muttered. He got the cordless phone dialed the number from a card stuck to the metal fridge door under a plumber's advertising magnet and slapped two pieces of white bread together with a dab of yellow mustard and three slices of turkey. "Ed Szabo returning a call from Bill."

He waited half a minute, taking a bite. With a mouthful, a voice came into the earpiece. "This is Bull."

"Ed Szabo," he mumbled through his sandwich.

He hesitated. "Mr. Szabo?"

"Yes."

"Your wife is not doing well today. She had an arrest several hours ago when we were trying to wean her from the ventilator. It took us a while to bring her back. I'm afraid she has not woken up yet."

"Should I come in?"

"It's your decision but she's stable for now."

"I'm not sure when I can get there."

"The intensivist wants to talk to you."

Food and drink in hand he hustled back to his garage and drove, indecisive about where to go. He ended up at the underground garage of the courthouse.

Chapter 44

By the time Ed arrived on the fourth floor and entered the double doors, Ramussen was asking Dr. Neville about her training and experience. As she flaunted her credentials for the audience, Hart waved impatiently to him to join him at the table. Judge Bradford looked displeased.

Hart's strategy to have two expert witnesses with the weakest testifying first appeared to be working. The diminutive gnome peering out of glasses too large for her face rendered most of the arguments levied by the team of defense attorneys against Grainger impotent. Her speech pattern, much like she had marbles in her mouth, and her undulating volume captivated the jury. Ramussen pulled details from her to keep her on the stand and on offense until afternoon recess. After more than an hour, he began to conclude.

"Dr. Neville, please summarize your position about referral to a center of excellence in heart failure."

"Older physicians such as Dr. Harrison often feel they may have the knowledge and ability to manage heart patients well and resist referral to those with the focus and additional expertise. However, the knowledge base in this area has double three or four times in the past twenty years. In recognition of this certified specialization in heart failure requires a great deal of additional education and training. In a city this size there's nothing to prevent patients from receiving up-to-date, cutting-edge care, as long as they are referred."

"Thank you, Doctor. I know you've been on the stand for a while but I would like you to conclude your testimony with a clarification of use of cardiac stimulants in patients such as Mrs. Thompson."

"This is a highly technical area and quite difficult for most physicians to fully embrace, let alone the lay public. As I mentioned, it takes additional years of education and experience in order to acquire a high level of expertise in this topic. Our facility provides outpatient treatment with dobutamine with excellent improvement in symptoms of heart failure. We use it judiciously in inpatients as well. The dosing and regimen used for Mrs. Thompson was not the standard of care in our facility or any others that I know. The rationale of withholding it as long as her symptoms were not accelerating was appropriate. However, the steep decline in her measured cardiac function, her ejection fraction as we say, called for a change in treatment. In our institution, low-dose dobutamine might have been given at some point to delay the need for mechanical cardiac support."

"How would you have treated her?"

"We would have done a heart biopsy probably around day 5 to 7. The defense argues that no benefit for a biopsy has ever been established in clinical trials. I would posit that treatment needs to be individualized and that a tissue diagnosis in this case would have resulted in a more rapid transfer and one life saved. Guidelines are generalizations not necessarily best for every patient. Mrs. Thompson's management was botched."

Several in the jury subtly nodded assent. Harrison jotted on his white pad.

"Why do you believe the patient should have been transferred earlier?"

"It is an assumption of mine. While Dr. Harrison used unproven therapy, certainly not established at the time he used it, he appears to have a reasonable grasp of heart failure. It seems logical that when faced with the diagnosis of giant cell myocarditis, an untreatable disease only diagnosed by biopsy, he would have transferred to a facility where she could get a cardiac transplant. He failed to biopsy. He mentioned referral in a latter note, so I think it is not a stretch to reach this conclusion."

"Is it your opinion that the delay in referral to a center where she could have received a transplant contributed to her death?"

"Without a doubt, yes."

Harrison continued to scribble, struggling to make it legible.

Jessop studied faces in the jury box and did not like what she saw.

"Do you think her outcome would have been better had she been transferred on Saturday?"

"While that was later than optimal, her chances of survival would have been drastically better if she had been moved on Saturday, when her decline was apparent. The dramatic deterioration that occurred later on Saturday and into Sunday would have resulted in earlier placement of a left ventricular assist device, a cardiac support machine not available at OCHA that would have saved her life. More accurately, I think she would have had an eighty to ninety percent chance of survival if she had been moved no later than Saturday. Her chance of survival at the time she arrived at Wasatch was less than five percent. It would have been a miracle."

"There was no miracle that day," Ramussen said. "Is it your opinion that either or both of the cardiologist defendants were guilty of malpractice?"

Two attorneys flew to their feet. "Objection!" echoed loudly in the chamber.

Dr. Neville's head nodded yes but she was prevented from speaking by the pandemonium.

"This calls for a legal conclusion from the witness," Stan Henriod called out.

"Sustained," the judge said. "The witness is instructed not to answer the question."

"Sorry, Your Honor," Ramussen apologized with poorly feigned remorse. "Let me rephrase. Is it your opinion that either or both of the defendants provided care that was below the current and acceptable standards of care?"

"Both of them did."

"I have no further questions for this witness." He watched faces as he returned to Ed's side and sat noiselessly.

Henriod held up a finger, asking for a moment of delay as he whispered with Jessop and Parr, deciding who would go first.

Judge Bradford announced, "It's about time for recess. Reconvene at two-forty." A gavel slap made it official.

The defense team minus Blackstone, who had wandered away with his wife, met in an adjacent room, arguing about order and strategy. Harrison went over his notes with Jessop while Pope listened in.

"That approach comes too close to shifting the blame to Blackstone," Pope interrupted.

"I won't go there," Monica stated. "You have to admit that this expert left that door wide open."

I'm going to have Frank crossing her first. He'll have a good chance to close it."

Pope rubbed the bridge of his nose rested without removing his weightless glasses, making them bob. He spoke to Henriod, then left the room.

"Are you confidant about your time estimates, Dr. Harrison?" Jessop asked.

"We used to do biopsies at OCHA but stopped years ago when the data did not support it. There's not a shred of objective evidence that a biopsy helps the vast majority of patients, despite what she or other experts claim. Admittedly, in this case, a rarity, it could have been. However, when you consider the length of time it takes to get a result, it would have made no difference."

"I hope so," she said.

They walked out together.

"I get the impression that if I get something wrong, I will be ripped to shreds and you will lose."

"If you neutralize the two experts, all you have to counter is the emotional component, the death of a mother in her prime."

"That's like saying if you want to run a four-minute mile, all you have to do is run the first three laps in under three minutes," she responded.

Before her sentence ended, they reached a cameraman waiting in the hall. "Dr. Harrison," a blonde woman reporter, tall and well dressed, called out. "Are you the physician who is behind the whistleblower claim?" She pushed her mic in his face.

Jessop stepped in front with one hand up. "We cannot comment on an ongoing case."

The reporter and cameraman followed them. "I'm referring to the case filed in federal court just after noon today," she clarified. "Are you the Dr. Hugh Harrison who is the whistleblower?"

Jessop pulled his arm and towed him back to the conference room. "I have no idea what you are talking about," she claimed.

The hall was too crowded to allow the cameraman to stay or get ahead of them. The attention of all those nearby was grasped by the small fray. Hugh opened the door for Monica, whose free hand dragged him with her inside.

The woman did not stop asking questions. The door closed.

"What was that all about?" Monica asked.

"I'm involved in a *qui tam* against OCHA. It was filed today, apparently."

"A whistleblower case? Did you tell me about this?"

"A while ago."

"OCHA is a codefendant here. Couldn't you have waited until this trial was over?"

"It's not exactly my decision. It's this firm from San Fran."

"Higgins Cowen?"

"Yes."

She muttered to herself. She pulled out a couple of pages of notes. "Give me a few minutes to look at these but stay here, if you could, in case I need clarification." She sighed, nervously fingering her crucifix.

Harrison sat, checking his watch.

He had to make a break for the restrooms before the recess ended and time was getting short The reporter was waiting for the door to open. When it did, the red light went on and the microphone went hot. "Are you the Doctor Harrison—"

"Please refer your questions to Higgens Cowen," he repeated several times to each question.

Inside the courtroom, Harrison was free of the harassment. The gavel sounded and Henriod approached the diminutive expert who was again on the stand and under oath, who appeared confident and superior. "Doctor Neville, was it a certainty that Mrs. Thompson would have lived if she had been transferred to a heart failure hospital on Saturday?"

"I did not say it was. I believe I used statements of probability. As you well know, little in life is certain."

"So, your answer is no."

"Yes."

He paused. "Yes?"

"Yes."

"So, your testimony is that it was certain she would have lived if she had been transferred earlier. Is that correct?"

"That is not how I answered."

"I think we are all confused."

"I believe you are the only one confused here, sir. You asked if my answer was no, to which I replied, 'Yes,' an affirmative to only that question. Perhaps you should rephrase."

Most of the jury smiled at the exchange. "You testified that you use dobutamine in heart failure patients, is that correct?"

"I use it in some patients, that is true."

"Is it a drug that is useful in heart failure?"

"When used judiciously, in the right circumstances and dosage, it is quite helpful in alleviating symptoms of fluid excess and improving urine production when diuretics alone do not have sufficient effect."

"It also makes the heart pump more blood, correct?"

"Yes."

"On the day Mrs. Thompson was transferred to the intensive care unit at OCHA, was her heart pumping a normal amount of blood?"

"No. Her cardiac index was 2.2 liters, as I recall. That is below normal."

"What is normal?"

"2.5 liters or higher."

"Do you recall what her first measure of cardiac index was after the dobutamine was started?"

"I believe it went up to about 2.5."

"That is exactly correct. Is it your opinion that this improvement was because of the drug?"

"Yes."

Half a dozen people in the court were thinking, hoping that he would stop right there. "Is it your testimony that dobutamine was helpful for Mrs. Thompson?"

"No."

"That seems at odds with your previous answer. Please explain."

Pope and Jessop exchanged glances, shaking their heads. Pope rolled his eyes.

"The initial dose used was reasonable but Dr. Blackstone kept increasing it. This harmed his patient. As with so many medications, it is not simply about the drug, it is how it is used."

"What a moron!" Blackstone whispered in anger.

Some of the jurors looked in his direction, as did Hart and Szabo.

"Did your client make a remark?" the judge asked.

Henriod shrugged.

Neville continued. "Within hours of excessive dosing, she began to deteriorate. With no hospital protocol and poor nursing education it is not surprising that a poor outcome occurred."

Parr began to object but he realized that he had no basis.

"That's quite enough, Dr. Neville," Henriod interrupted. She reacted as if slapped.

He attempted to wallow through a few more questions but stopped quickly, realizing he needed to get her off the stand as soon as possible.

Chapter 45

Jessop approached for her cross-examination, notes in hand. She did not like it but she could not remember the technical details of Hugh's questions.

"Do you recall the first left ventricular ejection fraction done on Ms. Thompson?"

"Yes."

Monica smiled confidently at the jury. The witness was being cagy and Monica relaxed.

"What was it?"

"The report said 45 to 50 percent."

"Did you review the study images, Doctor?"

"Yes, I did."

"Do you now agree with that estimate?"

"It's close enough. Yes."

"What is a normal ejection fraction by echocardiography?"

"Above 50 percent."

"Do you do heart biopsies, Dr. Neville?"

"Yes."

"How many do you do, say, in an average year?"

"Several hundred."

Monica took a moment to read from her pad. "Most of these are on transplanted hearts, I would assume. Is that so?"

"Indeed it is."

"How many times in the past year or two have you personally performed a biopsy on a patient with acute heart failure, such as Ms. Thompson?"

"This was an unusual situation which is infrequent and—"

"How many, Doctor Neville?"

"Maybe two or three."

"One?"

"Perhaps. I don't keep track."

"And that is at the Cleveland Clinic, a famous center with a large number of heart failure patients. Why so few?"

"We seldom see patients that early in the disease process. They are referred to us for transplant."

"When you do a biopsy, how long does it take to get results back from the pathologist?"

She blinked for a moment. "It's usually two days."

"Two days?"

"Two or three."

"In your practice, when you submit a biopsy on Thursday afternoon, when do you get the result?"

She squirmed. "Usually on a Monday."

"Do you have pathologists at the Clinic that provide this service?"

"Of course."

"Does OCHA have pathologists that provide cardiac biopsy pathology?"

"I doubt it. It requires a dedicated cardiac pathologist and specialized techniques."

"So, back to the ejection fraction. Would you have done a biopsy based on the first ejection fraction?"

"No."

What was the second ejection fraction?"

"Around 40 percent."

"It was 42 percent. Is that second ejection fraction, measured by a different method one day after the first a reason for a biopsy?"

"No."

Jessop studied her notes, pacing toward the jury box. "Is it clear that the second ejection fraction was actually different than the first, given the different techniques?"

"It is not clear that a change had occurred."

"Would you biopsy a heart with that ejection fraction, a native heart, not a transplant?"

"No, I would not."

"She had a third ejection fraction measured on Monday, April seventeenth, measured during a cardiac catheterization. Do you recall what it was?"

"As I recall it was 38 percent."

"In terms of impairment, is that mildly, moderately or severely reduced?"

"That is moderately reduced."

"In your entire career, how many times have you biopsied a native heart with an ejection fraction of about 38 percent?"

"Probably never."

"Is it your testimony that a biopsy should have been done when Ms. Thompson's ejection fraction was 38?"

Neville's mouth moved several times before any sound came out, the attention of all jurors riveted on her face. "Perhaps not."

"Perhaps? Would you have a biopsy?" Jessop faced the jury, watching reactions.

"I would not have done a biopsy at that point."

"Moving on to the fourth ejection fraction, done on Wednesday the nineteenth. It was done using the same method and technique as the second measurement. The number had dropped from 42 to 35 percent. Is it unusual to measure heart function so often?"

"It is. That is a lot of ejection fractions in a week."

"Four of them in six days. In your opinion, was Dr. Harrison attentive to the patient?"

She paused again, the question not anticipated. Her hand moved to her hair in her first nervous gesture. "It appears so but it is hard to state that with certainty since I did not witness the interactions."

"He had a complete note every day, wrote orders daily, followed her cardiac function like a hawk. How can you be uncertain based on the objective data in the chart."

"Being concerned and attentive does not negate that he was not taking good care of the patient."

Jessop thought about her answer as she turned again to the jury and put a soft smile on her face. "That was a double negative, Doctor. Maybe a triple. Would you like to try that again?"

Two jurors laughed out loud, earning a scowl from the bench.

Dr. Neville squeezed a smile on to her face. "It's looks like he was very engaged in her care."

"Thank you. So, now that Ms. Thompson had an established trend of decreasing heart function, would you have performed a biopsy at this point?"

"Yes."

"Please review the published evidence of benefit for this procedure with the jury."

"As I believe I testified, there are no publications that support clinical benefit from having a tissue diagnosis."

"So, it is your *opinion* that a biopsy would have been helpful. I believe you stated that earlier."

"Yes."

"Would it be reasonable to have an opinion that differs from yours?"

Again she hesitated. "Yes, but in this case, a biopsy may have hastened referral to a heart failure center of excellence."

"Is that based on retrospective information? That is, because she was found later on to have this uniformly fatal type of myocarditis which is quite rare, you believe that despite the utter lack of evidence of benefit, she should have been exposed to a procedure with risk?" Jessop stood close, bent a little to get at eye level and emphasized key words.

"Yes, that is my opinion."

"Opinion without a basis of fact, as you just testified." Jessop walked toward the jury box, referring quickly to the yellow sheet. "Do you know if OCHA had equipment for a heart biopsy?"

"I do not know."

"We will hear testimony later that they did not and do not have the device used to bite off small pieces of heart muscle. Do you know how long it takes to get a biopsy forceps?"

"If it is ordered early enough in the day, it could probably be overnighted by mid-morning."

"If Dr. Harrison had decided to biopsy Ms. Thompson at OCHA, it could not have been done until the following day, Thursday, correct?"

"That is probably true."

"What time on Wednesday was the ejection fraction reported?"

"I have no idea."

"Let's look." Jessop found the report and showed it to the expert. She studied it for a minute.

"It was dictated at one-thirty and transcribed at three-fifteen."

"In your experience would this be early enough to review the results, discuss the findings with the patient, schedule the procedure in the laboratory and send a purchase order for the required material to do the test?"

"It would be tight. I am not the right person to ask about specific timing at Olympus."

"I understand. If you learned at four in the afternoon that your patient needed a biopsy, would you do it that day?"

"It would be the following day."

"Once again, Doctor, a biopsy done at your facility in Cleveland on a Thursday afternoon would be reported to you when?"

"Objection. Asked and answered."

"Overruled."

Neville's jaw fell slightly. She looked left and right. Again, her jaw started moving. "Uh, I'm not sure." Jessop stood with the jury, waiting. "A routine study report would not come until Monday," she said with resignation. "However, a rush study could have some results available late Friday or early Saturday."

"And that would be at the Cleveland Clinic, not at OCHA, where the tissue would need to be sent across town. In light of this, can you honestly and with reasonable certainty say that a decision to biopsy Sarah Thompson made late on a Wednesday afternoon would have resulted in tissue diagnosis before she deteriorated on Saturday?"

"It's possible."

"But you just testified it was not likely. How can you fault Dr. Harrison for this issue, a procedure with risk, no established benefit and where the results would likely not be available until Monday?"

"If she had been in a heart failure center, these delays would not have occurred."

"Really? Okay, imagine that he had referred her late on Wednesday," Monica paced, speaking impatiently. "She would have been transferred on Thursday. The physicians would have seen her and possibly though not certainly, decided she might benefit from a biopsy that would have been scheduled on Friday with results still not available until Monday. How can you possibly say that the biopsy would have had a favorable impact on her outcome?" She positioned herself immediately before the witness, hands on hips and head cocked.

"If the information had been available in a timely fashion, I maintain her life may have been saved."

Jessop spun to face the jury. "If. How many of us say, 'If only'? Outside of the ivory towers, the rest of us must consider the world of reality. What else did Dr. Harrison do wrong?"

"Well, his choice to use a beta blocker was in error."

She went quickly to the table where the evidence introduced lay. She picked up a piece of paper and brought it to Dr. Neville. "Are you aware of this small study?"

"It is a small trial of the use of carvedilol in myocarditis."

"The trend was for benefit, correct?"

"It was not statistically significant."

"Were you aware of the study prior to today?"

"Yes."

"Why did you not reference it in your written report?"

"I did not think it was germane. The study was so small and done in Germany."

"So you wanted to hide it from us?"

"No."

"It is the only randomized trial that deals with the very heart of the allegations against

Dr. Harrison and you thought it was best to omit it. Do you think your decision indicates bias?"

"I am not biased."

"Then, explain for us in plain English how to rectify your failure to cite or even reference this study."

Neville was clearly uncomfortable. She removed and cleaned her glasses.

"We're waiting," Jessop stated.

"I misstated something earlier. I was unaware of the study until today. I did not find it when I prepared my report."

The judge cleared her throat and picked up her gavel, waving it subtly in indecision.

Neville glanced up at her under eyebrows tented with fear.

"It surprises me that a national expert in heart failure was not aware of this study until we provided it for court. How can that be?"

"It was done in Europe and the publication is obscure."

"What, Europeans can't conduct research?"

"Yes," she said.

"So despite the only study of carvedilol in myocarditis showed it cut the mortality rate in half, do you still claim that Dr. Harrison erred in administering this same effective treatment to Sarah Thompson?"

"Yes. It was not the standard of care then or now."

"Perhaps he has higher standards. How much do you get paid for your testimony?"

"I don't think I need to answer that."

Jessop looked up at the bench.

"You most certainly do," the judge directed.

"Six hundred dollars an hour for testimony."

"I believe it is more than that."

"Okay, six-fifty."

"How much for today?"

"Around five thousand dollars."

"Well, that seems to provide context to your opinion." She dropped her notes heavily on the defense table. "I have no more questions."

Dr. Neville stood to leave. The attorney for the hospital stood and approached her. She scowled and sat back down, likely longing to be back in Cleveland. As the cross-examinations dragged on her professional demeanor waned and vindictiveness grew.

CHAPTER 46

Ed and Amy made their way to the intensive care unit. Myra looked much worse. Small strips of tape intended to hold her eyelids closed had come loose so that her eyes were slightly open. Ed saw they pointed off in different directions. She stunk of sweat and vanilla. A mechanical forest of poles, pumps and tubing was on one side of the bed. A quiet console with an array of displays and controls was on the other. It connected to plasticized rubber pipes where water mixed with spit blew back and forth with each breath. Brown fluid oozed from the corner of her mouth and made a glistening trail to a puddle on a white towel under her neck.

"Where's Grandma?" Amy, in a hooded sweatshirt and jeans, looked at the person in the bed, swollen, misshapen and malodorous.

Ed pointed. Amy cocked her head and wrinkled her nose.

A nurse was looking over the IV pumps. He was almost six feet tall with muscular arms. His scrubs could not hide his small waist, sculpted thighs and chest.

"Hi, Mr. Szabo," he rasped. "Have you spoken to Dr. Pennington?"

"Not today."

"Hi, cutie." The nurse smiled, revealing gaps between his square peg teeth.

Amy snuggled up to Ed, shy and afraid.

"I'm Bull, your grandma's nurse."

Amy didn't move.

Bull rose to his full height. "I'll call the intensivist. She's probably still around." He left with large strides.

Ed pulled a pair of tissues from a box on the bedside table and wiped Myra's chin. He straightened the sheet, never changing his facial expression. "Oh, Myra," he said sadly.

"Myra." Amy, for the first time, spoke her name, not her title. She placed her compact hand on Myra's puffy forearm. Her face was also blank. She looked up at Ed. "Smells bad."

"It's what happens when you're in the hospital for a long time." He put his hand on top of hers and eked out half a smile.

The big nurse came back flexing and stretching. "Dr. Pennington will be here in a minute. She was just leaving." He took a sip from a bottle that said "Protein" in bold letters, then rolled his head around on his massive neck.

"My wife has been here a while but I don't think we've ever met," Ed said.

"I'm sorry. My name is Bull." His nametag said "William." He grinned. "At least, that's what I've been called for years.

"You are big enough to be called that."

"Oh, I've lost twenty-seven pounds in the last month or so."

"Really? Why?"

"I'm getting ready for a show this weekend."

Ed looked like he expected clarification.

"I have to lose skin fat so the muscles show better." He lifted up his left arm, flexed his bicep and forearm and tugged on the skin with his right thumb and forefinger. It was parchment thin. "It will be just about right by Friday night." Individual muscle strands and striations were already visible on the inflated extremity.

A gaunt wisp of a woman in a dwarfing white coat entered. "Hello," she said. "Pennington" was embroidered in pink on her jacket. Black rubber tubing looped out of one pocket. "I had thought you would be her sooner."

"I was in court," Ed said.

They shook hands. Pennington stooped at the waist, a forced happiness above her neck, hand extended.

"I'm Dr. Amanda. How are you?"

Amy tried to melt into Ed's side again, withdrawing, fearing the long, boney fingers. She did not answer.

"A little shy, are we? That's okay. It's a scary place here." She straightened to her full height, about the same as Ed.

"She looks worse," he said.

"We were trying to get that tube out of her trachea this morning. She seemed alert and lucid. We all thought she understood what was going on. When no one was looking, she pulled the tube out. The hospital won't let us restrain hands anymore, a policy that leads to stuff like this. At any rate, she did okay for almost an hour then began to tire. She couldn't manage her secretions. She quit breathing and we had a heck of time getting her re-intubated."

Amy relaxed her grip on Ed, who had nothing to say. Pennington walked around to the other side of the bed and looked up at the black monitor screen filled with numbers and lines.

"She was without enough oxygen for a while. We gave her a little bit of relaxing medicine and some sedation at the time but nothing since then. It looks to me like she had some brain damage. A neurologist will see her in the morning."

"So, this was an accident?"

"No. She just failed to wean."

"She has failed every day and this never happened."

"She extubated herself this time. Maybe it was her way of saying she's had enough of all this."

"Maybe it was a combination of dangerous policies, a hypoglycemic nurse and a mentally impaired patient."

Pennington said nothing. Hearing no response, he continued.

"You said you did not agree with the hospital's restraint policy. Nurse Bull said he had been losing almost a pound a day, obviously starvation. I'm not interested in covering up problems with some fiction about what you think she wants." His voice was even and tired.

"I'm sorry you're upset, Mr. Szabo." Dr. Pennington squeezed some words out.

"I'm tired and I do better with unvarnished truth. What's done is done. Let's move on." He reached out and touched her sleeve. "Where do we go from here?"

The IV pumps and the breathing machine noises became more intense in the conversation void.

"We wait for the neurology evaluation," she said.

"Thanks for talking to us," Ed said.

Pennington fidgeted for a moment then left. Ed's attention went back to Myra. He caught a drop of speckled saliva in a fresh tissue and pulled her lids down. Amy's hand returned to Myra's arm. Bull puttered with linens, the bed and the monitor.

"I heard your daughter died here a few years ago."

Ed nodded.

"I can't imagine how you feel, back here now with your wife so sick. That's gotta be hard."

"Never should have come back to this hospital. Aside from the bad memories, we're suing it. Did you know that?"

"Everybody knows and we're trying extra hard to make sure everything goes well. The problem this morning might cost the day nurse her job. She got royally reamed."

"I'm sure she did her best. Shit happens. Like I said, I don't do sugar coating."

Stan and Stacey Blackstone sat before a gas log fire, reading from the Old Testament.

"This section from the end of First Kings to here in chapter six in Second Kings gives me hope for this trial," Stan said.

"I thought today was good. Hugh's attorney in particular seemed to make a difference. She is quite pretty."

Stacey had a long narrow face and plain looks. Stan waved dismissively.

"Some chapters back, Elijah brought down fire from heaven when he was competing with the five hundred false prophets of Ba'al, consuming an offering, the altar, the Blackstones, the dust and the water he had poured over it all. Then he slew them, hundreds of men, single handedly. Later, he was protected from the law of the land as the Lord killed three groups of fifty soldiers when they came to apprehend him. Now, here is Elisha, surrounded by another army including horses, chariots and a great host. There is no way out. His servant, seeing the predicament, thinks death is certain and asks, 'What are we to do?' Elisha asked the Lord to open the young man's eyes and he saw the army of God in chariots of fire surrounding them.

"Where are you going with this, Stan?"

"I hear Elisha's words. 'Fear not: for they that be with us are more than they that be with them.' Stacey, I will prevail."

"I can't help feeling nervous."

"This trial is a distraction, a lot of noise. Elijah, again, said the God did not speak in an earthquake or in the wind. It was with a still, small voice. I can hear it. These false and malicious allegations will be blown away as chaff before the wind. I shall prevail."

"What about Hugh Harrison?" Stacy closed her Bible over a finger to keep her place.

"I don't think he has any hope for God's protection. He is a damned atheist and a dangerous doctor. He messed up this patient and scores of others. God shall smite him again. Our group nailed him in our suit and this will add to his punishment."

"You should do good to those who spitefully use you. Love is the answer. I don't like hearing all this anger from you."

"You're right, I should. It's so hard when he stole our money for years and stifled my career."

"Look around you, Stan. We haven't suffered much." She pointed slowly at the fine furnishings surrounding them.

"I'll try to return good for all his evil."

Stacey raised her eyebrows and looked at him over her reading glasses. The twist of her head said volumes about her skepticism. Stan failed to see it. The pleasant Bible session ended with a tale of two mothers boiling and eating a child.

Chapter 47

Malpractice Trial: Day Three

A little before seven in the morning, Dr. Pennington walked into the intensive care unit of OCHA Hospital, with a paper cup of coffee from 7/11, feeling well rested and ready for work. The nurses were gathered in the central station at shift change, talking hurriedly, pressed to leave or delaying getting started, depending on which end of the shift they faced. Typically the charts she sought were not in the assigned slot but with the teams doing the handoffs.

Bob, a short prematurely graying nurse, waved as he spotted her. "Are you ready for good news?" Bob asked.

"Always," was her reply.

"Mrs. Szabo is fully awake," he said.

"You're kidding me."

"Let's go see."

From the doorway they saw her, sitting up doing the morning crossword puzzle. Myra tried to look over but was tethered by the tube in her mouth. Her hands were restrained and though she tried to bend down and reach up, she could not adjust the traction to allow her to see. Pennington and nurses entered and moved into her field of view.

"Good morning, Myra," Pennington greeted.

She waved with her pencil.

"She's been on CPAP since about four, breathing on her own," another nurse, Mahindar, reported. "Thirty-five percent oxygen, no 'pressors."

"You look great. How do you feel?"

Myra put a pad of paper on top of the newspaper and wrote her response. "Fine. Please take this tube out, <u>PLEASE</u>." She underlined the last word half a dozen times.

"I've got to look at your bloodwork and X-ray first. But this is the best you have looked since you came in here."

"BS" a written response.

The trio left.

"I don't understand how that happened," Pennington said as they walked.

"I think she may have been over-sedated yesterday," Mahindar suggested.

"Great," Pennington groaned. "Another screw-up on a litigious patient."

She whispered an assortment of profanities through gritted teeth as she looked at all lab reports and other tests. Bob was getting far too much enjoyment from the interaction with the lovely goddess-nurse.

Ed's home phone recorded the brief call me back message while he was again in court.

Doug Thompson strutted out of jail that morning wearing jeans and a T-shirt.

Dennis Hart's secretary met him at the door. "Thanks," he said.

"Don't thank me," she said. "Follow me."

Little else was said as they found Hart's silver Mercedes.

As they drove, Doug squirmed, then spoke. "How did Mr. Hart get me out?"

"Never mind how. He needs you in court."

"Is that where we're going?"

"We need to make a stop at our office. Would you object to a haircut?"

He shook his mane. "It has taken me years to grow this."

"Yes or no?"

"Will it help us win?"

"Mr. Hart thinks so or he wouldn't do this for you."

"How about a ponytail?"

"Haircut you win, ponytail you lose."

"How's it going in court?"

"Our experts testified yesterday and did a lot of damage." She was sincere because she was not present. "We have good momentum and a great plan for today. Haircut?"

"How short?"

"Not very. When we're done you'll look like George Clooney."

"Yeah? Well, good luck with that. Are you going to cut my hair?"

"Only if you want to win this case."

"Even if we win, I'll still be in jail."

"But you could hire the best defense team in the country."

"Okay, then."

After parking, Harrison went to the entrance of the courthouse and hit speed dial for Dominici, hoping he was not on West Coast time. He had been called half a dozen times in the last hour. Reporters wanted interviews. He tried to be polite the first time, tried to be firm the next. He simply hung up on the last three callers. His call went to voicemail. "I need some guidance about how to handle the press. Call me." He then reentered the building and to the elevator.

"What in the hell do you think you're doing?" Parr confronted Harrison as he entered the large noisy hall from the elevator.

"I beg your pardon."

Parr moved close. He was an inch or two shorter than Hugh but at least seventy pounds heavier. "Your *qui tam*, you scumbag. It's in the news right in the middle of this trial. Have you lost your freaking mind? It could make everyone lose, including you."

"I had no control over when it was going to be filed."

"Don't give me that crap," he grimaced and raised a clenched fist with one finger pointed at Hugh's nose. "If members of the jury heard this, actually, when they hear it, it will create the impression you're at war with the hospital."

Harrison twitched when he was hit with spittle. He wiped his face. "Which is true." "Which neither of us can afford."

"Zone should have considered that before breaking the law."

Parr backed off after looking around, straitened his tie, smoothed his cheap suit. "Listen, Doc. I only have to defend the hospital. This morning they asked me to change strategy. We're siding with Blackstone, defending him and the hospital."

"That's the OCHA I know and love. Does Pope agree with throwing me under the bus?" He shrugged. "You'll be so deep in debt, the only way out will be a bullet to the brain."

Jessop approached. "What's going on here? You look upset, Matt."

"Did you hear that Harrison is the whistleblower in a claim against OCHA and Chandler Cardiovascular?"

"And Parr just threatened to kill me."

"What!" Jessop's voice echoed in the hall.

"I did no such thing."

"Bullet to the brain is not a threat?"

"Stop! Take a breath, both of you." Her eyes bore though Parr.

"Filing a claim against your codefendant in a multimillion-dollar lawsuit is reckless," Parr said.

"Dr. Harrison, don't you think you should have given us a heads-up?"

"I had no idea when it would be filed until it was in the news."

"Zone's going to the mat against you," Parr said.

"Everyone gets dirty in a mud fight, Matt," Jessop said.

"Well, that's the tricky part. And by not waiting 'til this is over, you guaranteed your loss."

"Not my decision."

"No wonder your ex-partners hate you. You're a damn weasel."

Franklin Pope, attorney for the liability company, had appeared out of the crowd. "Good morning, all," he intoned in a mellow baritone. "Pejoratives are the sound of unhappiness."

"Do you know about the qui tam?" Parr asked.

"Just found out this morning."

"The hospital wants Matt to hang it all on Dr. Harrison," Jessop said.

Pope rubbed the bridge of his nose with advancing discomfiture. "We can't afford to let emotions spill over from that turbulent sea into ours. There's a lot of money at stake here. We cover both physicians, a real balancing act in this case. We would like a win for both of them. If we cannot, my company would rather have one payout than two. We'll see how this plays out from here but if it's clear there's a winner and loser, our efforts shift to the winner."

"Nothing like a little more pressure," Monica said.

"Who would you rather have lose?" Harrison asked Pope.

"I don't care. If both of you lose big, we pay $2 million. If one loses, we pay $1 million."

They filtered into the room along with the rest of the small crowd. Parr went straight to

Henriod, who was trying to settle Blackstone down. As he whispered in his ear, Henriod's brows went up.

The gallery had grown. When court convened, a barely recognizable Doug Thompson sat at the table, shampooed, cut and styled and in a nice suit. A few wisps of gray around his forty-year-old temples added an appearance of success and sophistication. His tattoos were not visible. After Ed got past his initial surprise, he spoke in a manner Doug would understand. "You dress up good."

"Did Hart bring in another attorney?" Blackstone asked Henriod.

"It looks like the ex-husband got out of the slammer and cleaned up for court."

The judge welcomed Mr. Thompson, who nodded politely. Hart started the day with the heart surgeon at Wasatch who had operated on Sarah. He testified she was practically dead on arrival but was loathe to lay any blame. He had a long and friendly acquaintance with Harrison plus he depended on cardiologists to send him business, as Henriod pointed out on cross-examination.

Hart then called the nurse who attended to Sarah during the shift when she crashed, Jason Jeppson. She had entered the cardiac ICU talkative and comfortable. At the end of his shift she was on life support. Blackstone had seen her, placed the monitoring catheter and started her medications, then did not return when she deteriorated despite several phone calls, documented in his notes. Blackstone left the ICU management to Dr. Malloy. Jason knew of no policy for dobutamine in heart failure patients. His testimony took an hour. After recess, Jessop established that Blackstone provided all the care that day and that Harrison was never contacted. Parr took a few minutes to establish the quality and oversight as well as the fact that Jason had additional help in the ICU from a highly experienced nurse when he needed it.

Henriod took his turn last. "Mr. Jeppson, do you understand what myocarditis is?"

"More or less."

"More or less, then, what is it?"

"An inflammation of the heart."

"How does one get it?"

"I don't know."

"What is the treatment?"

"I don't know."

"These are things that a typical nurse may not know but that a cardiologist would know, correct?"

"Yes, sir."

"How many patients with myocarditis have you taken care of in the cardiac intensive care unit?"

"Only one that I know of. That was Sarah."

"So, given your lack of experience and knowledge, which is not unusual for most nurses, do you have any factual disagreements with the care rendered by the two defendant physicians?"

"No factual disagreements, no, sir."

"Do you have a good relationship with these two cardiologists?"

"I hope so."

"That's all I have for this witness." Henriod returned to his side of the court and Jason looked at the judge, wanting to be dismissed.

"Redirect, Your Honor?"

"Go ahead, Mr. Hart."

"Jason, do you have any disagreement with the care given by Dr. Blackstone in particular that may not be factual, just your opinion?"

"The choice of medications is not for me to judge."

"I'm just asking about your concerns, that's all, son."

"Well, I was shaken at how quickly she tanked. I mean got sick so fast. I thought it was not best that Dr. Blackstone would not come in but had Dr. Malloy take charge. Dr. Malloy is very good, great in fact. But he is not a cardiologist and her problem was cardiac."

"Would you send one of your family to see Dr. Blackstone?"

"I object," Henriod stated. "Irrelevant."

"It addresses the relationship and trust between this nurse and Dr. Blackstone, which Mr. Henriod addressed with his final question on cross-examination."

"I'll allow it. Overruled."

"That is a very uncomfortable question."

"I know. I'm sorry." Hart waited.

Blackstone's face prickled.

Jason looked at the jury, biting his lower lip. "He would not be my first or second choice," he said hesitantly.

"If this close relative were in the care of Dr. Blackstone, would you be comfortable and confident that he or she would receive the very best care?"

Henriod strained to keep quiet. Judge Bradford helped out by frowning at him. Jason adjusted his tie and collar and shifted in the wooden chair.

"That is potentially a very uncomfortable question. I have to work with Dr. Blackstone and would prefer not to jeopardize our working relationship."

"That is a sufficient answer, Jason. I appreciate your time and your choice to be a nurse." Hart faced the jury. "People trust nurses more than they trust attorneys, which is not saying much."

Laughter.

"They also trust them more than they do doctors." He turned back to the judge. "I have no more for Mr. Jeppson."

Rosa directed her gaze at Henriod, who was already getting to his feet. "I have another question or two of this witness, Your Honor."

She waved her hand in permission.

"Did you ask Dr. Blackstone to come in?"

"I don't specifically remember. I told him she was doing poorly and was struggling to breathe. His response was for me to call Dr. Malloy."

"And you did, correct?"

"I told Dr. Blackstone it was his job to speak with consultants, not mine. I got Malloy on the phone and they talked."

"So, Dr. Blackstone took action based on the information you called to him but you did not request his presence?"

"I wanted him to come in. Normally, doctors come in when there is a significant deterioration. But I don't remember specifically if I asked him to come in."

"I'm going to accept that as a 'no.'" Henriod sat. "No more questions."

The judge allowed Jason to leave.

The bailiff called a Charles Rockwood, a forensic accountant, to the stand. Hart rubbed his hands as he was sworn in.

Judge Bradford shuffled a few papers, adjusted her bifocals and peered over them at the clock. She asked, "Would the defense like to call its first witness before lunch? It appears we have time."

"Yes," Parr said. "The defense would like to call Jennifer Hayes, vice president of OCHA Hospital."

Hayes appeared in a dark wool suit and little jewelry, appearing to be the consummate female executive. Her nursing background and practiced demeanor gave an impression of caring competence. It did not take long for this witness to lay out a string of quality awards and treatment protocols used for Sarah Thompson. It was an impressive list.

Early in cross-examination Hart handed her a paper with a fresh evidence sticker. "Here is a list of the local hospitals, Jordan River, Sandy Heights, Good Samaritan and others including OCHA, Ms. Hayes. Next to each hospital is a list of awards. How many awards do you see listed for each?"

"Between two and ten, Mr. Hart."

"Have I left any hospitals in Salt Lake valley off the list?"

"No." She pursed her lips and raised her brows.

"So if every hospital wins awards, no one is truly distinguished, right, Mrs. Hayes?"

"It's the difference between winning a dog show at the American Kennel Club or the Tooele Depot Dog Display, Mr. Hart."

Several jurors chuckled at the local humor.

"Or maybe like becoming Miss Kamas Rodeo or a Victoria's Secret Model."

More laughter earned a look from the bench, although the squat judge was herself amused.

"Our awards are from highly esteemed organizations."

The reference to underwear drew Hart's eyes to Hayes' neck and cleavage. The expression on his face did not change but he walked closer. "I want to ask you about your hospital's protocols for heart failure."

"We have the highest ranking in heart failure management," she interrupted.

"I haven't asked you a question yet, Mrs. Hayes."

"I am so sorry, Mr. Hart. I thought you did. I thought trials were about bringing all the facts to light. Perhaps not?"

He referred to his yellow pad. "Do you have a written protocol for heart failure management?"

"We have order sheets and several assessment tools that constitute a protocol, although it is not labeled as such."

"So no formal protocol?"

"Our protocols are codified as order sets."

The dual continued until Hart seemed to give up trying to discredit the witness or her institution. Court was recessed.

Sandwiches had been delivered to the Hunter Hinkley & McKay firm, where Jessop and Henriod practiced. Pope, the liability company attorney, had arranged and paid for the meal.

As Harrison was about to enter, Pope snagged him. "I need to ask you and Dr. Blackstone to stay out for a few minutes as we try to sort out this mess you created with the *qui tam*."

Harrison saw Jennifer Hayes inside, towering over Stan Henriod, speaking with her best open-face look, but still failing not to be overpowering. "Sounds reasonable," he said.

Jessop brought out a turkey and cheese sandwich, then went back inside. When Blackstone arrived, Pope had a quiet conversation with him as well.

"I think I'll take a walk," Harrison told Pope as he was closing the door, leaving the two cardiologists alone together in the waiting area. "I'll see you back in court."

"You might want to stay here and defend yourself. It is bound to get harsh."

"Parr already threatened assassination. I'll take my chances on the street."

"I'm sure it was a figure of speech in a heated moment. Just stick around. Jessop will call your cell when things calm down."

"Good luck with that." He left as Henriod brought Blackstone some food.

Inside the room there was a hum of small talk and arguments. "Everybody just settle down," Pope said. "I talked to the attorney who filed the whistleblower suit, Dominici, an hour ago. They made it part of their strategy to file while our case is in court. The publicity and timing serves their interest."

"At our expense," Parr muttered.

"Agreed. But it's done, no pulling it back. So, we need to focus on winning this case, not on retribution. Are we clear?"

No one answered.

"So, Frank, you sit in the gallery every day, watching the jury," Hayes said. "How do you think it's going?"

"Hard to say since we haven't had a chance to present a defense."

"We would prefer to hang this on Harrison and protect Blackstone."

"I'm not getting in the middle of any vendetta."

"Like you said, Frank," Parr said, "if both docs lose, your losses could double."

"True in the short term. I could make a better argument for putting it all on Blackstone." Frank looked tired. "He's had a flurry of claims and they keep coming. He is part of the twenty percent of docs that burn eighty percent of the premiums. We have settled three in the last two years. A loss here will give us no choice but to drop him."

"If he lost a million here, would he be over the lifetime coverage limit?" Henriod asked.

"He would get close to the $3 million limit. One more small award or settlement and he would no longer be insurable with any of the standard carriers."

"He can't practice at ICHA without insurance," Parr said. "He'd lose his job."

"The man needs more of an intervention than we've been able to muster," Pope said.

"He has a strange detachment," Henriod said. "A kind of surrender of responsibility or something."

"If you need to take sides, Harrison must be the one to pay," Hayes repeated.

"It's not your decision, Jennifer." Pope put his hands in the air. "I understand your agenda but you are not paying the bill. My first goal is to defend both successfully. My second is to minimize my losses."

"Harrison is taking us to court," Hayes argued. "We're going after him here and now, regardless of what you want."

"Oh, be rational," Jessop said.

"It is imperative that we behave as a team," Pope said "If Harrison loses big, a lot of that money could come from you."

"Chump change compared to our losses if this ridiculous federal claim gains traction.

We need to bury his ass." Hayes was visibly angry, her face flushed.

"You need to cool off," Pope said. "Let's get through this afternoon and reassess where we are after three or fours of defense testimony."

"I think that's reasonable," Parr said to Hayes.

"It's not best for us, Matt."

"Any other comments?" Frank directed his question to Jessop and Henriod.

They shook their heads.

"Let's get the docs in," Henriod said.

"Harrison took a walk rather than spend two seconds with Blackstone," Jessop answered.

"Can you blame him?" Parr, Pope and Henriod said almost in unison, followed by laughter.

"Damn!" Henriod exclaimed. "I'm late. I need to pick up our expert from the Hilton." He dashed out, tie flapping in the wind.

"Get Blackstone in here," Pope said. "We need no outbursts in court."

CHAPTER 49

"Hi, Dr. Harrison." It was not a male voice that answered Dominici's phone. "Tony was going to call you but something came up."

"Lisa Jacobs?"

"Yes. As you know we filed."

"And I have reporters pestering me."

"And we went over what to say to them."

"No comment and that's it?"

"It's a case in litigation and your counsel prohibits you from commenting on it."

"That'll look good on TV."

"Try to look noble. And refer them to us. We decided that Melissa will do the media. She has the Utah look, blonde, blue eyes."

"Why file while in in the middle of a lawsuit?"

"OCHA and your partners are both in the local news, not that it's covered much so far. By naming them now, the trial publicity should increase and the guilt by association helps us."

"And mine, too?" Hugh was irritated.

"We think you could skate."

"You have more confidence than I."

"The jury, along with most everyone else, will find you more likable than Blackstone."

"Seriously?"

"Millions of dollars are on the line, Doctor. We do our homework. How's the trial going?"

"We're just starting our defense," Hugh offered.

"So, maybe a verdict by late tomorrow?"

"Maybe that soon. I doubt it."

"Call as soon as you can when it's announced."

"Won't you know?"

"Probably, but we'll need to connect on strategy, depending on the outcome."

A cameraman and a TV reporter watched the defense team exit the elevator and walk into the courtroom. Harrison was not with them. The reporter caught a glimpse of might have been Harrison sneak into the courtroom from a stairwell.

"You know what," the reporter said. "Why don't you go back to the station without me? I think I'm going to watch some of this malpractice trial." He entered and sat in the gallery.

"This is Dr. Maurice Djamdjian," Henriod announced to the team assembled at the table before the judge's entrance was announced. "He's our expert from New York. This is Dr. Stanton Blackstone."

The bailiff called, "All rise!"

Within minutes, Djamdjian was sworn in and on the stand. Henriod approached. The dwarfish doctor with a moderate Armenian accent possessed a soporific voice and a nervous tic of nose scratching.

Education, training, publications, job history were presented in the usual fashion. He fell far short of the two experts hired by the plaintiffs, one of whom, Dr. Paulette Neville, was in the gallery immediately behind Hart and next to Ramussen. Neville had laptop and typed intermittently.

Henriod guided the expert through the days of hospitalization. The time of day combined with the dreary lack of inflection and boring subject matter tended to put people asleep or close to it.

Pope signaled with a rolling index finger to speed up. Henriod shrugged in return.

Blackstone issued a few sonorous breaths, then issued a loud snore. Parr nudged his shoulder, causing a loud snort followed by a ripple of suppressed laughter. Judge Bradford straightened up, opened her eyes and looked around to see what was going on. Parr shook Blackstone's shoulder with more vigor until his eyes flipped open.

Henriod looked over his shoulder as Djamdjian droned on about the chemical structure of dobutamine and the shape of adrenergic receptors where it stuck and altered intracellular flux of calcium, potassium and sodium and the actin-myosin interactions. Pope drew a thumb across his throat when Henriod cast a glance in his direction. He brought the testimony to a halt. A recess was called.

"Nice snort," Harrison quipped as he rose from his chair.

"Go to hell."

"Boys, no fighting," Jessop warned. "Certainly not in here." He was second from the aisle.

Henriod had already exited but Blackstone was not moving. She put her hand gently on Blackstone's shoulder to urge him toward the exit. "Don't touch me," he growled as he twisted and knocked her hand away.

"For the love—! Move so I can get out, then," she said.

He didn't move. "How can you live with yourself, defending this douchebag?"

"Just move," she answered.

"He is pure evil."

"Oh, brother!" Monica said to herself.

"Brother? You said brother? Like Cain and Able maybe and he," Blackstone raised his voice and pointed at Harrison, exiting the opposite direction, "is pure evil."

"Please, sir, keep your voice down," the bailiff said.

"Take a hike," Blackstone sneered as he spun on his heels and started toward the double doors at the rear.

"Hold on, sir!" Blackstone kept walking.

Jessop reached out to the bailiff. "He's stressed. He'll settle down after a little break."

"He'd better," he said, hoisting his belt and squirming his neck.

Jessop caught up with Harrison, who was waiting at the door. "That was a little weird," she said.

"He is all that and more."

"I thought he was religious."

"He is. I wonder how bad he'd be if he weren't."

"You know him pretty well?"

"Better than I'd like."

"Is he mentally stable?"

"I'm not a shrink. But, he makes me nervous."

On the other side of courtroom, Brett Rasmussen, Hart's junior associate, had watched the interaction between the two physicians. A few minutes later as they walked to lunch, he asked, "Do those two docs hate each other?"

"Probably."

"Are you going to leverage that?"

"Only if it makes both of them lose."

CHAPTER 50

Hart stood to begin the cross-examination, teeth sharpened, thoughts focused. "Where did you grow up, Doctor?"

"Armenia."

"I'm confused about your résumé. You list two medical schools, one in Armenia and one in New York. Did you flunk out of the first?"

"Hardly. I graduated with honors then joined my family in New York City. None of the hospitals there accepted my medical training so I could not get an internship. I had to repeat school all over again in this country."

Hart faced the jury and made a dismissive "humph." "Let me cut to the chase here, Doctor. Is it your testimony that both of these two cardiologists provided appropriate management of Sarah Thompson for the period in question, despite the dramatic differences in treatment?"

"I believe I stated earlier that neither of them did anything wrong."

"That is not what I asked."

"It was an appropriate answer for your question, sir."

"I don't think so. Did both Dr. Harrison and Dr. Blackstone adhere to the standards of care for Sarah Thompson?"

"There are no published guidelines specifically for myocarditis. I believe they cannot be faulted for failure to adhere to some imaginary rules. To find them in noncompliance would be akin to giving a traffic ticket to someone for jaywalking on a country road where there are no crosswalks."

"If you had a patient such as Sarah Thompson, whose heart function was deteriorating as rapidly as was hers, would you refer her for advanced therapies such as transplant or a ventricular assist device?"

"Specialists in heart failure are readily available in the hospital where I practice and I would defer to them."

"But Dr. Harrison did not refer her, did he?"

"In a sense, he did. He called a heart failure super-sub-specialist."

"But he did not send her. When she finally arrived at Wasatch, the cardiac surgeon testified she was virtually dead on arrival. That implies that Dr. Blackstone transferred her after she had deteriorated beyond the point of salvage, does it not?"

"I believe it is not sound to reach that conclusion."

"Virtually dead on arrival and you can't decide if the transfer was too late?"

"In the hospital where I practice, ventricular assist devices are available. When you need to transfer across town, I imagine the logistics take extra time. Some things may be outside the control of the physician. There can be no bed available for the patient, for example. It is not a simple black-and-white situation, sir."

"If you worked in an environment such as OCHA, would you not learn to compensate for such vagaries?"

"That depends on how often such an act occurs. If you transfer patients on a regular basis, one would know how long it takes and make the necessary adjustments. I don't know how often OCHA patients *in extremis* are sent to Wasatch."

"We, the public, trust you physicians to make correct decisions in life-and-death situations, do we not?"

"Yes, sir."

"Sarah Thompson had such a situation and died, didn't she?"

"She did."

"On a more-likely-than-not basis, was it more likely that she would have survived if she had been initially admitted to your hospital?"

"It's impossible to say."

"Was it more likely she would have survived if she had been admitted initially or electively to Wasatch?"

Djamdjian removed his glasses, pulled a handkerchief from his pocket and cleaned the lenses and replaced them on his face, adjusting them carefully as the breathing in courtroom slowed. He looked at the defense table, into five pair of eyes. Hart went to speak but the expert lifted a hand. "It's a good question, a probability estimate. Unfortunately, we are forced to view it retrospectively and through the emotional veil cast by an untimely death. This makes it quite challenging. One must separate the emotional issues from whatever science and data exist. There are a lot of variables to consider, so many unknowns. To be perfectly honest, I don't think the answer can be known with certainty."

"I'm not asking for certainty," Hart said. "Her chance of survival, was it better at Wasatch with all the tools and expertise available or at OCHA where resources were limited?"

"At the cardiac center, of course. She was sent there for that reason."

"Yes, where she arrived almost dead, a couple of days too late, correct?"

"She was close to death when she arrived there. That is not a debatable point." He held eye contact with Hart.

"That wasn't so difficult now, was it?" Hart said, then walked around in silence for a moment, letting that exchange settle into the minds of the jurors. "Doctor, you spent a lot of time in your testimony talking about dobutamine. You seem to know a lot about it."

Djamdjian did not answer the implied question.

"Would you and others consider you an expert on this drug?"

"Yes."

"For the jury then, please can you cite one study, or more than one if possible, where dobutamine in the dosage used on Mrs. Thompson had a beneficial effect on death rates in heart failure patients?"

"I am not aware of any trial that shows a convincing improvement in mortality."

"Mrs. Thompson was treated with dobutamine at a high dose, correct?"

"In an effort to keep her alive until she could get advanced support."

"Dr. Blackstone failed to keep her alive that day. Both doctors failed the patient by not sending her to Wasatch." Hart's pitch had gone down but volume up, his voice ringing like a death bell, echoing in the solemn chamber and his finger pointed at the defense table, where Dr. Blackstone recoiled. In fact, most of the people jerked in pain. "And you somehow think that was okay?"

Djamdjian's head pulled back, Hart's righteous face glowing not two feet away, like Moses parting the Red Sea. "It was a tragedy."

"It was a lethal comedy of errors," Hart growled through clenched teeth. He stood straight again and tugged at his suitcoat to restore the fine drape of fabric. "Is it your sworn testimony that dobutamine did not and could not have contributed to the untimely death of Sarah Thompson?"

"There is no reason to believe it contributed to her demise."

"I thought research was clear. Dobutamine results in an increase in death rates."

"The tiny increase in mortality rates was reported in patients with chronic heart failure, not acute as was the case here. The deaths occur later, not during treatment. There are no data for people like Mrs. Thompson."

Most of the jurors had perked up at this exchange.

"Does that mean this drug could not have hastened her death in the dosage Dr. Blackstone used?"

One bead of sweat coalesced on Djamdjian's scalp, made a stuttering decline down his forehead, then dripped into his lap. He pulled out a brilliant white handkerchief and dabbed his pate. "There are no data, so an answer would be speculative." Hart folded his arms, waiting for more.

Djamdjian unhooked his wire rims from his small ears, removed his glasses, patted his eyes and swept beneath his nose. As he reattached his spectacles he spoke as their eyes locked on one another. "The drug is commonly used to support a failing heart and that's how it was used in this case. It's a standard practice."

"Can you tell the jury that you have a high degree of certainty it did not make her worse?"

"While I don't think it contributed to her deterioration, I cannot truthfully testify that it could not possibly have made her worse."

"You moron!" Blackstone's chair legs screeched as he shrieked and stood, shaking his fist at the witness. Henriod and Jessop pulled him down but not before he screamed, "Idiot!"

"Order!" Judge Bradford called on top of Blackstone's epithet as she fumbled to find her gavel. "I will have order. Mr. Hemorrhoid, control your client!" The name faux pas brought poorly stifled guffaws from the gallery. "Order!" She slapped the wooden mallet thrice hard on her podium.

Harrison saw Ed with a huge smile, something few people ever witnessed. Ed chuckled silently and soon had to wipe a tear from his eye. The judge called several times for silence and order was restored.

The Honorable Rosa Bradford in her impeccable English spoke. "Dr. Blackstone, another outbreak and I'll find you in contempt of court. Is that clear?"

"Yes, Ma'am."

Henriod nudged him. "Stand up and address her as 'Your Honor,'" he whispered.

Stan did so as she glared at his lack of decorum. "Mr. Hart, do you wish to continue your cross-examination?"

"I have no further questions, Your Honor."

The Judge looked at the defense table. "We need a short recess, Your Honor, just ten minutes," Jessop requested.

"Good idea." She popped the gavel.

The jury paraded out and the gallery emptied.

"Dr. Blackstone, do you have any idea what you just did?" It was the rumbling voice of Franklin Pope.

"You call that idiot an *expert*? He was killing me."

"It would not shock me if you paid $2 million for each of your three words."

"Where did you find this guy?"

"We've been over this, Doctor," Pope said. "We went through over a dozen potential experts until we found one that supported both of you. It wasn't easy. Let's get out of here."

"You just damaged your defense," Henriod said. "You can't blurt out insults at the expert who is defending you and expect to win."

"I'm not sure we can recover from that," Pope said. "I think we should offer five hundred thousand to settle for each of the docs. That's a million total. They might go for it. It'll save the company a million."

"You want us to make them that offer?" Jessop asked. "After that, I'm pretty sure they'll laugh us out of the room."

"Damage control," Pope said. "Arrogant doctor, a boring expert, a dead mother, an impaired child." He exhaled loudly. "I smell a multimillion-dollar verdict."

"I am not arrogant. He was an imbecile." Stacey Blackstone, standing nearby, shook her head. Her eyes met Harrison's briefly before she quietly left the room.

"Is it okay with you if we settle for that amount?" Jessop asked Harrison.

"I won't settle now."

"We're on the ropes," she said.

"I've got 'em where I want 'em."

"Oh, God." She frowned before she couldn't help smiling.

"You don't have a choice," Pope said. "Neither of you do. You gave us permission months ago to negotiate a settlement."

"All you guys do is settle," Blackstone said. "I should look for a different malpractice insurance carrier."

"We're not the only game in town," Pope said.

Blackstone was taken aback.

"Stan," Pope directed, "propose a total settlement of a million dollars on behalf of the doctors, five hundred K for each doctor."

"How much for the Chandler Clinic?"

"Same."

"That's generous, Frank," Henriod said.

"I'll follow suit," Parr said. "Half a million from the hospital. Total settlement $2 million."

"That's a huge number for a settlement," Jessop said.

"Go," Pope said.

Henriod and Parr left.

"I really don't like this," Harrison said.

"Legal malpractice," Blackstone said.

"If it weren't for your big mouth in the first place we'd never be here." Pope pointed his boney finger in Blackstone's face. "And you did it again! What will it take for you to control your tongue?"

The break was over and jury was seated but the bailiff ushered them out again. The judge was giving time to the ad hoc settlement conference. It didn't take long.

Henriod joined his team shaking his head. "Not going to settle at this point," he said.

"Put Hayes on the stand, Matt," Pope said. "That'll give the rest of us time to revise strategy."

"Both your docs are killing us," he said. "In very different ways."

Near the end of the cross-examination of Jennifer Hayes, the group of attorneys reentered.

When Hart sat, Henriod announced, "We would like to call Dr. Blackstone."

Parr whipped around and looked at Pope, who remained impassive. "What the hell are you doing?" he whispered.

"We need Blackstone's testimony as far from the end of the trial as possible," Jessop whispered back after Blackstone had placed his hand on the Bible.

CHAPTER 51

Blackstone had planned on objecting to the swearing in process on the basis that it violated his religious rights, compelling to do something that was proscribed in the Old Testament. He did not. He searched unsuccessfully for Stacey in the crowd. The plump and reddening Stan Henriod quickly extracted his training, credentials, work and personal history. Hired by Dr. Harrison in 1994, fresh out of cardiology training at Loma Linda University, he had quickly become a successful cardiologist by the time he took care of Sarah Thompson in April of 2004.

"How did Dr. Harrison communicate information about Sarah to you?"

"I can't recall exactly. We always provide a printed list of our patients for the guy on call for the group on weekends and put some notes about what has gone on and what to do."

"Did he speak with you about his patient list?"

"Probably but I don't remember. We usually do."

"For how many cardiologists did you take call on a typical weekend that year?"

"Four."

"How many patients did you see that weekend?"

"I saw fifteen to twenty patients that weekend."

"Is that a lot?"

"It's pretty average."

The petty and boring details of the weekend were presented to the jury along with his vague recollections of Sarah. The examination ended late in the afternoon.

"Mr. Hart," Judge Bradford called. "It's late but we still have about half an hour. Do you wish to start your cross-examination?"

"I do indeed, Your Honor."

"Proceed."

He came forward with a covered poster, placing it so both the jury and the witness could see it. He removed the cover with a slight flourish.

"Do you recognize Ms. Thompson?" There were portraits of four women about the same age. "Can you point at her from this array?"

He became desperate, studying each face. "Well, Dr. Blackstone?" Hart was tapping his foot quietly but audibly, looking back and forth between the jury and his prey.

"It's not a fair question," he objected. "When I saw her she was ill, had no makeup, no combed hair. Most of the time she had tubes coming out of her mouth and nose."

"So, you don't recognize Ms. Thompson from these four women. There's a blonde, a redhead and two brunettes, one of whom is very dark. There is short hair and long hair. I might add, she had not changed her hairstyle from when this picture was taken."

He studied the poster carefully, his bowel starting to rumble. He moved his right forefinger between portraits, targeting. "I'm not sure."

"Please, take a guess."

Stan pointed at the blonde, who looked like an accountant should look, Teutonic and bookish.

"Let the record show that Dr. Blackstone pointed at Mary Jo Hart." He looked at the jury. "That is my lovely wife," he said with a smile.

"Bottom left," Harrison said quietly.

Hart ignored his comment. The photo array was introduced into evidence.

"Dr. Blackstone, you do educational seminars and other activities to maintain your license every year, do you not?"

"I do."

"When was your last educational event this year?"

"It was in March. I attended the A.C.C. meeting, the annual Scientific Sessions of the American College of Cardiology."

"Do you get certificates for the educational events you attend?"

"I do."

"You produced your continuing medical education papers as a part of the discovery process prior to trial. I would like to introduce them into evidence now." He lifted a thin sheaf of documents from the corner of his table and brought them to the recorder who marked them. "Take a look at your educational history from 1994 to 2004, Doctor. Please show to the court where you had education specific to heart failure."

Blackstone's mouth opened and his eyes blinked blankly at Dennis Hart before he looked at the papers. He shuffled slowly through as Hart waited patiently. "I attended meetings about interventional cardiology. I didn't attend any seminars specifically on heart failure; however, the topic is covered throughout other talks and topics."

"No education on heart failure in general. Did you get any education dealing directly with myocarditis?"

"No."

"Why not?"

"It is a rare condition."

"Rare? Really?" Hart wheeled with a finger in the air and pawed through a stack of papers, extracting one between finger and thumb. "Is Schwarzwald a reliable textbook of cardiology?"

"Perhaps the best."

A chapter from the book was introduced as evidence. Hart handed it to Dr. Blackstone.

"Would you please read out loud this part highlighted in yellow?"

He read it.

"What percent of young people who die from accidents or similar causes have myocarditis?"

"It says around one percent."

"So, do you wish to stick to your statement that this is a rare condition?"

"What I meant was that rarely do we see people as sick as this patient was."

"So, if this is such a rare event and your focus is not heart failure, why did you not send

Ms. Thompson to a heart failure center sooner?"

"I, uh—" Blackstone closed his eyes and bowed his head for a moment.

Hart as well as people in the gallery and jury began to stir uncomfortably until Blackstone spoke.

"Dr. Harrison didn't send her. I tried to do what he wanted until it was clear she needed help we didn't have."

"He told you he didn't want her to refer her out?"

"Correct."

"When Mr. Henriod," pronounced distinctly as *Henry Odd*, "asked you if Dr. Harrison spoke with you about Sarah, you couldn't remember. Now you remember?"

"Yes, er, no. I'm not…." He went silent.

"Please, Doctor, answer the question."

"I'm not certain how I had the impression that he wanted the patient to stay in OCHA but that affected my decision to keep her there."

"The patient?"

"Yes, the patient," Blackstone snapped.

"You are talking about Sharon Thompson?"

"Of course."

"Or Susan Thompson?"

Henriod and Jessop exchanged looks of horror. Harrison put a hand over his eyes and shook his head. Ed, seated at the plaintiff's table, rolled his eyes.

"Sharon. Mrs. Thompson."

Hart let that sink in. Speaking in the direction of the jury, he said, "Did you tell Sarah, yes, that was her name, and her family that you thought Dr. Harrison did not have her best interests at heart, that you were going to take the bull by the horns and get her on the road to recovery?"

Blackstone pondered. "I may have said something like that. It was three and a half years ago and I don't remember exactly what words I spake—spoke."

"Did you want to establish that you superior, that you could offer better care than Dr.

Harrison?

"I didn't need to prove it."

"Because you already knew it?"

Behind Hart, Jessop and Henriod were exchanging silent, angry words about client preparation, objections and old-fashioned name-calling.

"I didn't need to prove anything."

"Why did you communicate to Sarah's family that your partner was not, shall I say, fully engaged and doing what was best?"

"She had languished in the hospital for eight days deteriorating. I wanted to stir things up, the waters of Bethesda, you know."

"That's a reference to a story in the New Testament, is it not? One of healing a cripple."

"It certainly is." Blackstone sat up a little taller. "I'm impressed that you are familiar."

"This is a religious city, Doctor."

"Perhaps, but not one that knows the Bible well."

Hart raised his eyebrows so the predominantly Mormon jury saw. The last statement would infuriate some of them.

"Did you have a close, collegial, positive relationship with Dr. Harrison at this time?"

He thought with his eyes closed. "We were partners at the time."

"I was asking about your professional interactions. Were you good partners?"

"He did his work his way and I did mine. We covered call for each other, so it was functional."

"He left the practice shortly after this, correct?"

"Yes."

"Why was that, Doctor?"

"That's a better question for him."

"Did he tell you why he was leaving?"

"We never had a conversation about it."

"Why do you think he chose to leave?"

"He couldn't get his way anymore. He was no longer the big chief, just another little Indian like the rest of us."

"Were you happy to see him go?"

"Yes."

"Why?"

"He created discord. He took a cut of our revenue for himself. He had become a liability." Henriod loudly cleared his throat attracting the attention of everyone but

Blackstone.

"Stealing? How much money did you make in 2003?"

"I don't recall."

Hart paged through papers again and found the desired sheet. "Was it around $340,000?"

"It could have been."

"How much did Harrison make that year?"

"I don't know. I never had access to that figure."

"Would it surprise you if he made $30,000 less than you?"

"It would."

"That's the amount on his W-2. How much did you make in 2006, well after Dr. Harrison left the practice?"

"Again, I don't recall exactly."

Looking again at the data, Hart backed toward the jury box. "Does $820,000 sound close, Doctor?"

A few gasps arose from the both the jury box and the gallery.

"That could be close."

"Your income more than doubled after Dr. Harrison left. Was that because he stopped stealing from you?"

"Maybe."

"Why did your income go up so much after he left?"

"Objection," Henriod offered. "Irrelevant."

"Overruled. Dr. Blackstone opened the door, Counselor."

"Answer the question," Hart said.

"It was partially the income from our cath lab."

"The issue that was in the news this morning?"

"What news?"

Hart played to the jury again. "Maybe later. Did Dr. Harrison's departure have anything to do with your increased income?"

"Objection! Relevance and calls for speculation."

"Your Honor, this goes to the strained relationship between the doctors that affected the transfer of information and the care of Mrs. Thompson."

"I'll allow it. Overruled. Please answer the question."

"No."

"Did Dr. Harrison propose and supervise development of the cath lab?"

"Yes."

"Did he propose or support the contract with OCHA, the agreement that, according to your statement a moment ago, almost doubled your income?"

"Your Honor," Henriod stood. "Objection! This has gone far afield."

"Make your point, Mr. Hart."

"Answer, please, Dr. Blackstone," he said.

"He opposed the arrangement. After he left, we were able to complete the negotiations and make it happen."

"And make a lot of money, apparently. This opposition, as you call it, caused some disagreement between the two of you then?"

"Between him and most of us."

"Were you angry with Dr. Harrison in April 2004?"

"I would call it disappointed."

"Not angry?"

"I don't get angry."

"You don't get mad?"

"That's correct."

"So when you burst out earlier today at your own expert, calling him a liar, what would you call that?"

"I was simply pointing out his error."

"Not angry?"

"No."

"I see, I think. I had a different impression. I'm going to shift topics." He returned to his table. "In fact, this might be a good time to break, considering the hour."

"I agree," Judge Bradford concurred.

The court adjourned for the day.

Chapter 52

In the early evening, Pope called Jessop.

"Did you get Hart to settle?" she asked.

"If you think a total of $15 million is a settlement."

"We never should have put Blackstone on the stand, Frank."

"Yeah. The reason I called is that I had a conference call with Dr. Malouf and Jennifer

Hayes. Malouf told me if we didn't scapegoat Harrison, she was going to pull her entire group out and insure with a competitor. That's a large loss of premium."

"What did Hayes say?"

"That she would pull all of her employed physicians out as well. It would be an unmitigated disaster for us."

"I'm not sure we could possibly put this all on Harrison, given Blackstone's performance on the stand. Plus, personally I'd have a hard time throwing Harrison to the wolves. He's a class act, the kind of doctor we should want to clone."

"I've never had this big of a mess," Pope said. "If I lose that much premium, I'll out of a job."

"Please, don't ask me to sacrifice Harrison."

He sighed. "We'll sleep on it and meet at 7:30 tomorrow and try to come up with something. Christ, what a cluster!"

Early that evening Ed and Amy drove to the hospital after a stop at MacDonald's for Amy. They made their way to the ICU.

"It's about time you showed up." The unrecognizable raspy voice came from Myra, sitting in a recliner with a cup of water in her hand. Her white gown with tiny blue fleur-de-lis dipped wet and low on her chest.

"Grandma!" Amy shouted. "You're back!" She ran up to her and gave her a hug.

"You look much better than I expected," Ed said. "You were worse yesterday."

"They took that damn tube out early this afternoon and got me out of bed a few minutes ago."

"This is almost miraculous. I'm stunned, amazed."

"What day is it? I've lost track of time."

"You've been in the ICU for two weeks. It's Thursday, May 29."

"My God! That's a long time."

"We're in the middle of the lawsuit."

"Really? I'm missing the whole thing." That's what she tried to say. Her voice gave out.

She patted Amy gently on the back then sipped more water.

Jen, the ICU nurse, came in followed by Dr. Lester Malloy, the intensive care specialist.

They were both dressed in blue scrubs with "Property of OCHA Healthcare" stencils prominently displayed front and back, top and bottom. He had grown a ponytail since he had taken care of their daughter.

"Hey there," Malloy said. "It's Dr. Pennington's turn to have some time off, so I'm back.

She looks good, doesn't she?"

"I'm confused about how she looked so much worse yesterday and so much better today." Ed scratched the back of his head.

"We are simply grateful she has recovered so well," Malloy said.

"What did you do?" Ed asked.

"Edmund!" Myra croaked, almost inaudibly.

Malloy said nothing.

"We let all the sedatives and pain medicines wear off," Jen explained.

"That makes sense," Ed said.

Myra attempted to talk but just gasped and sputtered. Ed tugged at her drooping gown to pull it up, protecting her modesty.

"If she does well overnight, she'll be moved to a different floor in the morning, if there is a bed available," Malloy tried too hard to look optimistic.

"Sounds good. The over-sedation is resolved then?"

"I think she's a slow metabolizer, plus the drugs go into fat and heavy people might store up a lot."

"Most of us understand that mistakes happen. All of us are human. As long as the error is not flagrantly stupid we are not just capable of forgiving, we want to. A frank explanation binds us together in a way. But deception drives us apart."

"Ed, there you go again." Myra gasped.

"What about greed?" Malloy was unfazed. "Some people sue for millions of dollars when no mistake occurred."

"Our little Amy has spent the last three years motherless. Look at her. She will likely never be independent and will always require some financial support. Her mother provided that, not her father and certainly not us. If some egregious error caused Sarah's death, how does one seek remediation? Or do you think it's right that Amy pay for a preventable error that a doctor made?"

"Of course not," Malloy said.

"So, what happened to Myra?"

"She received too much of a drug the other night," Jen said. "An overdose. It was a nursing error. We figured it out and Myra got better."

"Thank you," Ed replied graciously. "Now that the truth is out, everyone can relax and feel better. Even you, Myra."

She glared at him but said nothing. She was struggling to breathe. The figures on the monitor were still all normal. Dr. Malloy left. Ed pulled up a folding chair and sat several feet away from his wife. Amy started playing with the bed controls.

"That was very nice, Mr. Szabo." Jen stood with folded arms surveying the family scene. "I'm not a vindictive guy." Ed relayed a summary of the trial.

Myra didn't offer her usual criticism and complaints, just pursed her lips and breathed with effort.

CHAPTER 53

After leaving the courthouse, Blackstone drove to his office. It was well after closing but Dr. Malouf and Cheryl Williams were watching as a team of federal agents boxed and cataloged Liles. Cheryl was the third practice administrator in as many years.

A male agent noticed Stan enter and faced him. "I'm sorry, sir. You can't come in."

"I'm Dr. Blackstone. I work here."

"Understood. This is a federal investigation."

"I need some medical articles from my office."

"Show me," the agent said.

Blackstone went to his office, the man following close behind. When he entered, he reached for a stack of work. "Don't touch, Doctor."

He asked another agent wearing blue latex free gloves to assist. He picked up the stack. "Is this what you need?"

"Yes."

He went through every page, a collection of papers on myocarditis and heart failure. He recounted the pages and handed the stack to Blackstone.

The gloved agent said, "These have nothing to do with the investigation."

The agent handed the stack to Blackstone and said, "Let me show you out."

Blackstone arrived shortly thereafter to a quiet home. Cinnamon spice candles were burning as Stacey was reading to four-year-old Rachel out of a bible stories for children book. He walked by without a word and found his study where he plopped down in a black leather desk chair and began swirling around, staring at the rotating ceiling. His papers lay on the desk untouched when Stacey came in.

"How are you?"

"You left this afternoon. Where did you go?"

"You upset me. I couldn't stand to watch anymore."

"What do you mean?"

"I don't think you realize how bad it looked, to stand up and scream at your own expert witness."

"He was lying, for goodness' sake! I could not stand idly by and let that go unchallenged."

"You don't get it." She exhaled in frustration.

"Don't be condescending on a day like this."

"If your fly were down, would you want me to let you know?"

"This is different."

"Maybe in your mind but not in mine. All I'm saying is that it looked terrible." She remained barely inside the doorway, shifting weight from one leg to the other. "The jury sees you differently tonight."

"Perhaps with more respect."

"No, Stan, more likely disdain. It's hard to understand how it is you can't see this. What's going on with you?"

"What's going on with you?" He spoke loudly. "Look at you. You're wearing pants! You left me in court! You're criticizing me!" He stood and threw both hands in the air. "I'm doing God's work." He glared at her through briary brows as she retreated. "But you, you behave like Job's wife, failing to stand by me, siding with my critics." She was well into the hall when he paused. "But you go ahead. I am a man of faith, strong, unwavering, unassailable," he shouted.

Stacy was afraid but did not leave. He continued to talk to her through the doorway. "Though I walk through the valley of the shadow of death, I will fear no evil. Thy rod and thy staff, they comfort me. But, rods and staffs are used to strike and harm. How would that comfort someone? Spare the rod and spoil the child. Your lack of faith, the false accusers, the selfish hospital and the godless Harrison all strike me with blows that comfort and purify, cleansing me in the crucible of the court. This balm of affliction soothes me, assuages my soul."

Stacey had seen him like this once before, when he was a medical resident and sleep deprived. He got help then and took medication for months. She was ready to run in case he came after her, as he had done then. But he dropped to his knees in prayer. "Surely goodness and mercy shall follow me all the days of my life and I will dwell in the house of the Lord forever."

Gliding forward, Stacey closed his door, giving him privacy and protecting his sanctum. Ten minutes later, she and Rachel careened out of the driveway in the minivan with suitcases seeking safety. Her family lived in Arkansas so they had nowhere to go that night but a motel.

CHAPTER 54

Jana and Harrison sipped coffee after a dinner of leftovers in her small condominium. Her cat, a splotchy mix of grays and black, nestled on his lap as an old foreign film, *Kiss of the Spider Woman*, with subtitles played on the old Toshiba television. He studied Jana's nose as she watched. From the front it had a classic Grecian appearance. From the side, there was a small flat area, almost a depression, in the middle where the cartilage took over from the bone, and one endearing unique little feature. She thought it was an ugly flaw.

She kept looking over at him uncomfortably. "Why aren't you watching the movie?"

"I can see it out of the corner of my eye." He smiled. "As if eyes had corners."

"Stop staring at me."

He ran a finger over her cheek, through the downy vellus hair, invisible except when close. "I'm pondering the whys of my attraction to you. Part of the answer could be in your pulchritude."

"What body part is that?" She crossed her arms over her chest.

"It's an attribute, not an organ."

"You and your words." She resumed watching as did he.

Her ears were small, tight and firm. Two pierced holes in the lobule he could see. "Your anti-helix is almost circular."

She rolled her eyes and shook her head. Her long thin fingers squeezed the remaining heat from her coffee mug. He got up and filled up her cup with fresh hot brew. She lifted the steam up to her imperfect nose and inhaled. "Mmmmmm." She looked at him. The tip of her tongue protruded for an instant beyond her teeth when she said, "Thank you." Her lips assumed a seductive shape at the end of the phrase. Her eyes remained on the screen until he sat again. She punched the pause button and focused on Hugh.

"You haven't said much about the trial this evening. Will it end tomorrow?"

"It will probably go to the jury in the afternoon."

"So, what happened in court today?"

"Our expert was annihilated on cross exam. Blackstone yelled at the end of the guy's testimony and called him a liar. Then he got on the stand and was shredded by Hart. It is hopeless. The jury is going to award so much money to this little girl it'll make national news."

"Are you sure you're not exaggerating?"

"I doubt it."

"Did you take the stand?"

"Tomorrow. After Blackstone's crucifixion is complete, I'll get nailed to my own cross." "Cut the drama, Hugh. It can't be that bad."

"Maybe not but today was a pivotal day in favor of the plaintiffs. It'll take a miracle to win. God and I are not on good terms, so I have little hope she'll go out of her way to cut me a break."

She laughed, as she usually did when Hugh spoke of God as feminine. "Whatever happens, things will work out. They always do." She grasped one of his hands and squeezed. "I'll still be your friend. It won't be a total loss."

"We should celebrate tomorrow night," Hugh suggested. A question formed on her face. "Why? Any number of reasons. If the award is a million bucks from me, it won't exceed my malpractice limits and none of the money will come from me personally. If the award is more, then we should spend money while we have it, because it will soon be taken."

"What if you win?"

"There is no winning, only escape. Tomorrow, Hart is either going to win big or accept a settlement of millions of dollars. I see no other outcome."

"We'll see."

There was a lull. Harrison left the couch to find a phone book when Jana hit play on the remote. The gay prisoner resumed trying to talk his straight cellmate into a liaison. He called Flemings, a steak house downtown, for reservations.

Jana paused the show again. "I'll tell you what, Hugh. If you lose more than a million dollars on this thing tomorrow, we'll terminate this celibacy thing and have sex. Pity sex. How's that sound?"

"Are you trying to make me testify on behalf of the plaintiffs?"

She laughed long and as loud. "No, you idiot."

"What do I get if I win, then?"

"You get to keep your house and car and your job."

"I think I'll take the loss."

She turned her attention back to the show. "Bonehead," she said when he sat next to her, put his arm around her.

They snuggled through the end of the flick.

"How was the trial today, hon?" asked Melanie Ramussen of her husband Brett as he walked into the kitchen.

"It smells good in here. Mmmm. It went well for us, I think. The expert for the defense was a true piece of work."

"How's that?" Melanie, an avid runner, asked.

"First he was boring as all get out. Then Dennis got him to support our side!" Brett was animated, not how he usually acted after a day of law. He looked like a golden boy, trimmed hair, clean shaven, square jaw, gym-sculpted chest. "It was laughable. Plus. PLUS! One of their docs started snoring during his testimony. *That* was priceless."

"Was it Dr. Harrison who snored?"

"Naw, it was Blackstone. He's one odd duck."

"So it went badly for Dr. Harrison."

"Indeed!" He smiled and rubbed his hands. "What's cooking?"

"He saved Brady's life."

"We've talked about this, Mel. This is my job, our income. It's not personal."

"Brady's your brother-in-law. My sister would be a widow if Dr. Harrison hadn't been there."

"Anybody would've done as much."

"Like Dr. Blackstone?"

"You may have a point there."

"Or Hatcher, who can't seem to keep it in his pants?"

"Where's this coming from?"

"Andrea. She's friends with one of the receptionists that works in that office."

"I should talk to her. Get some of the down and dirty, the nasties."

"She and Brady are coming over for dinner tonight. Should be here anytime."

That brought a pause. "Since when?"

"She called, we chatted, I invited them over. We haven't seen them in over a month."

"Why did she call?"

"What? I can't talk to my sister without giving a deposition?"

"Alright, fine. What's got into you?"

"We are having chicken and dumpling stew. One of your favorites."

The doorbell rang, then the door opened.

"We're here," chimed a familiar female voice.

A couple of hours later Brady and Andrea left.

"Hon," Brett said, "that was a great dinner."

"Thank you."

"And that was a most interesting inside look into a dysfunctional group of arrogant jerks. If it's true."

"So, what if Harrison was the victim of a mean-spirited campaign to eliminate the ethical guy, the one who made the rest of them look pretty mediocre or worse in how their patients did?"

"Too bad for him, Mel. Nothing I can do about it."

She just looked at him.

"What?"

"Do you really think he deserves to lose this lawsuit?"

"Mel, my job is to win."

"Seriously? Regardless of whether he's guilty or not?"

"So Brady thinks the guy walks on water. So Andrea worships him. 'I love that man,' she said. That's a bit over the top, don't you think?"

She looked away. Soon her eyes glistened.

"I got this job to represent our clients. Harrison's attorney does the same. The jury decides."

"Who replaced the kind, ethical guy I married with the heartless executioner?"

"I don't hand out the sentences. I advocate."

"If you really think the world is better off without doctors like Harrison, the guy who saved Brady's life, then go ahead and advocate him out of practice. Put scores of people at risk with less-skilled cardiologists just to make a name for yourself. Yeah, Brett, talk about a piece of work."

"Come on, Mel," he called after her as she ascended the stairs to the bedroom. No answer came.

CHAPTER 55

Verdict

First thing in the morning Stacey Blackstone went to their bank when it opened and wired as much money as she could to her father's account in a small bank in Norman Oklahoma. The banker warned her the transaction could be traced since movement of almost $900,000 would trigger an alert. He explained how to avoid the notice of the feds but she did not have time to do small, daily withdrawals or transfers. It was once her father's money, she rationalized, and it went from one of her accounts back to her father's with interest. A huge amount of interest. He was going to divide it between banks in the Bahamas and the Cayman Islands, undoubtedly triggering another alert.

She stopped in at her attorney's office and filed for divorce. If the award was not large, she could drop the legal proceedings, although it remained tempting to pursue regardless. Stan and she had grown in different rates and directions with increasing friction and decreasing compatibility. In this last week these factors overpowered the religious obstacle to the act she had pondered for years.

She entered the courtroom a little after 10:00 in the morning to find her husband screaming at Dennis Hart. Judge Bradford gaveled a recess at the hasty request of Henriod and Stacey left without saying a word. She felt his eyes pierce her back as the doors closed.

After lunch, Jessop addressed Harrison, the final witness for the defense. "Why didn't you refer Sarah to the heart failure clinic?"

"Two reasons primarily. First, it took five to seven days of observation to establish that her heart function was deteriorating. Secondly, patients I had sent to their institution were almost invariably enrolled in a clinical trial. Most of the drug trials done there were on stimulating drugs, all of which had negative results, meaning there was no benefit and sometimes harm. I'm a supporter of research but it made me hesitate when I had a young mother in my care. I was still holding out some hope that her deterioration would stop on the regimen I was using and from a symptomatic standpoint, she had not gotten any worse while I was taking care of her."

Jessop referred to the complicated graph Harrison had made of over a dozen clinical measures that covered the time of Sarah's admission until the Saturday when Dr. Blackstone assumed her care. At the demand of Pope she'd had an artist edit the graph to exclude the deterioration when Blackstone assumed care. The only graph that trended down was the left ventricular ejection fraction. They went over the graph for several minutes.

"Both of the opposing expert witnesses criticized your use of carvedilol, a beta blocker. Why did you use that drug?"

"Their criticism is understandable. It has been stated more than once in this process that there is no established medical treatment specifically for myocarditis. Beta blockers and particularly carvedilol are clearly beneficial for chronic heart failure. Neither of the two experts provided data that these drugs are were harmful in myocarditis because that data does not exist.

"It's common for physicians to treat conditions for which we have little or no research data. At that time and even now, there was no study that showed harm from the treatment I used. Today we can look at the one very small trial that suggested benefit, the paper that was introduced here a couple of days ago. It was too small and not well controlled enough to be definitive but it doesn't impugn my care."

Jessop studied the jury as he spoke. She spent more time looking at their reactions than she did with her witness. "Just a couple of items to cover before your cross-examination. I'm certain Mr. Hart will ask about any disagreements between you and Dr. Blackstone. Did you and he have a poor working relationship?"

"I was leaving the practice, so many of my former partners were upset. I didn't think it affected the practice arena."

"Thank you, Dr. Harrison. I may have more questions on redirect." As she passed the plaintiff table, she said, "Your witness."

Without standing, Hart fired the first question. His voice was hoarse and the words not clear.

"What was the question?" Harrison asked.

Hart took a sip of water, cleared his throat and rumbled, "Why did you leave the practice, Chandler Cardiovascular?"

"The values of the practice changed."

"Changed? In what way?"

"More of a financial emphasis than we had in the past."

Blackstone's chair squeaked as he slid back, ready to stand. Henriod put a heavy hand on his shoulder to hold him down and whispered something in his ear. Anger glowed in Blackstone's eyes.

"Making money is part of running a business or a medical practice. Can you explain your issue more clearly?"

"I thought some of our acquired cardiologists were overly concerned with revenue."

"Is this related to the so-called whistleblower suit, the complaint you filed with the U. S. attorney that has been in the news?"

"Objection. Irrelevant." Jessop stood as Hart remained seated.

"It addresses the relationship between the two defendants," Hart countered.

"It is prejudicial, Your Honor, and as a case in progress, inadmissible."

"In chambers, please." Judge Bradford stood to her five feet plus whatever heels she wore and disappeared to the rear of the room. Murmuring started as the two opposing attorneys made their way back.

Harrison stretched his legs, surveying the scene. Ed Szabo was looking at the jury. One of the jury, an older woman watched Doug. Doug was glaring at Blackstone, who in turn was rising from his noisy chair, eyes fixed on door closing behind the judge. Bloodshot eyes, day old stubble and tousled hair made him look mean. Henriod urged him to exit and seemed to make an effort to stay between the two physicians. They followed Jessop toward the rear door. Attorneys Parr and Pope lingered behind in quiet but intense conversation.

The bailiff escorted the jury from the room. Blackstone stopped suddenly and spun around Henriod, his teeth clenched.

"What's up, Stan?" Harrison asked, backing up.

"You have caused me nothing but pain for years." He advanced, fists clenching and stretching.

"I hired you, gave you a good job in a thriving practice. What's so painful about that?" Harrison caught a glimpse of Doug looking in their direction.

"God hath cursed you. People despise you." He continued to advance as Harrison backed up.

"Come on, Dr. Blackstone," Henriod said, pulling on his shoulder. "Stop it!"

"You deserve to suffer, to crawl on your belly and eat dust like your serpent master." With both hands he shoved Hugh hard against judge's pulpit. "Your punishments will get worse because you revile against all that is good."

Blackstone's left fist went hard to Harrison's belly. His right hand cocked but Thompson caught it and, with leverage, pulled it down over the parapet, catapulting Blackstone onto the floor. A few of the jury saw some of the altercation. Blackstone bellowed in pain, grasping his misshapen shoulder.

The bailiff turned and saw Thompson standing over a howling physician while the other doctor was doubled over, hands on his stomach, eyes bulging. He pulled his gun and aimed at Doug, screaming, "Hands in the air, in the air!"

"No!" the jurors yelled.

Doug put his hands up, high and wide as he undoubtedly had done many times before and fell to his knees before asked.

"What in the hell is going on here?" the old bailiff yelled.

Muttered profanity issued from the Man of God writhing on the floor.

Harrison loudly gasped for air. "Thompson," he choked out as he pointed, "was protecting me from Dr. Blackstone."

One onlooker said, "He caught the doctor's fist before he could throw a punch and pulled him over the wall onto the floor. He's the good guy here." He could barely be heard over Blackstone's screams.

"Stay put," the bailiff said to Doug, who remained on his knees. "Are you hurt?" he asked Blackstone.

He kicked at the officer. "You moron!"

"It's his shoulder," Harrison said. "Call paramedics."

The ruckus brought more onlookers into the room by now and the noise level rose. "My God, it hurts! He assaulted me, you idiot!" he screamed at the bailiff.

"Blackstone attacked me," Harrison managed to speak. "Doug stopped him."

The bailiff holstered his weapon and gestured with his head. Thompson stood. The bailiff called for back-up through the radio on his shoulder. Jurors were drawn back into the room by the commotion. The few remaining in the gallery pressed forward talking, asking, accusing. Blackstone continued to bellow in pain. Hart, Jessop and Judge Bradford all returned to witness the pandemonium. Jessop hurried to where Hugh was straightening up, hands over his stomach. Henriod stood over Blackstone, eyes on the ceiling, shaking his head in disbelief.

Hart tugged Doug aside. "What the hell was that?" he whispered.

Ed took a seat with a Zen-like half-smile on his face. Judge Bradford pounded with her gavel, calling for order and for the room to be cleared and the jury to exit. Half a dozen uniformed officers eventually filtered in.

The lawmen and women emptied the room. Within minutes a pair of firemen with medical kits entered and began attending to Blackstone, who would not stop his incessant whining. Paramedics soon followed. The tumult eventually died and the courtroom resumed its proper decorum when it was empty.

Chapter 56

"I should have gone to med school," Stan Henriod said as a dollop of mayonnaise oozed from his sandwich.

"You could have been the sui-ee instead of the sewer," Hugh quipped as the drop hit Henriod's lap unnoticed.

"Was that an attempt at a lawyer joke?" Jessop asked, stirring her noodle salad.

Four attorneys outnumbered the doctor at the table of a noisy Italian restaurant.

"It looks like this case is going to spill over to Monday," Pope was all business as usual.

"Bradford is probably livid."

"I don't know," Jessop replied. "If Hart crosses Dr. Harrison for under an hour, we'll have time for closing arguments and jury instructions."

"Not sure the judge will continue after that debacle," Parr said.

"She knows it will take under an hour for the jury to decide." Jessop sighed. "Then it's just finding out how many millions are awarded from whom."

"Is it too late to settle?" Parr asked Pope.

Pope shrugged.

"What did you do to Blackstone to make him come after you?" Henriod asked.

"The same reason he does angiograms on people. I have a pulse."

"Funny."

"He just came after me. Did I say something wrong when I was on the stand?"

Pope poked at his quesadilla, his shoulders slumped and face crestfallen. "We don't get a lot of choice about who we get to defend in this business."

"I don't remember ever having a trial this... entertaining," Jessop said.

"Blackstone likes you, Stan," Pope said. "He has requested you for his next dozen cases."

No one laughed until a slight smile broke on Pope's face.

"You need to learn to like him."

"He must be an acquired taste, though I admit my wife likes him." He paused. "And so do my banker and broker."

After a few chuckles Pope suggested, "We should make a motion for a mistrial. It'll be cheaper than filing an appeal."

"How many of the jury witnessed the fight?" Parr asked.

"Not sure," Henriod said. "A couple, I think."

"Why do your partners think you're a punching bag?" Pope asked.

"Never stand between a doctor and a dollar bill," Parr said.

"I thought that was a lawyer joke," Jessop said.

"Do us all a favor," Pope said, "and file charges of assault and battery. If he lost his license, we wouldn't have to cover him."

"That's the motto of the insurance industry," Harrison said. "Find any way not to pay claims."

Monica reached into her purse on the floor and pulled out a cell phone. "Hello."

This was followed by a brief series of acknowledgements and a "They're all here with me. I'll take care of it." She flipped the pink lid closed. "Bradford wants to see us in chambers in twenty minutes."

Pope waved at the server to get the check. "I'll bet she's thinking mistrial as well. It will keep her docket on schedule."

The meeting was brief and court reconvened on time. With the jury seated, the judge spoke. "We'll continue with the cross-expraction of Dr. Harrison. You are instructed to ignore anything that may have occurred after the morning session ended. Acts outside this trial are not germane to this proceeding. Okay. Mr. Hart, you may continue. Dr. Harrison, you are still under oath."

Ramussen stood. "Your Honor, Mr. Hart's voice is hoarse. He asked me to continue with the cross-examination."

Hart nodded. Bradford gestured to proceed.

"Dr. Harrison, you said you regretted not referring Mrs. Thompson to the Wasatch heart failure program, did you not?"

"I did not use the word regret in that context."

Ramussen rubbed his chin. "Your Honor, could we hear Dr. Harrison's exact words?"

Judge Bradford directed the recorder to read back the transcript, which confirmed Harrison's memory.

"Good enough," Ramussen responded. "Do you now regret not sending her to Wasatch?"

"Like I said, when you look back at things, they seem a lot more clear. I should have bought stock in Microsoft and Apple. I should have invested with Warren Buffet. I never should have married my first wife."

Several jurors laughed.

"Now that I see that Sarah died, I wish I would have done something different. At the time, I did what I thought was right. I have wondered if things would have turned out differently if I had transferred her instead of having Stan take—er, Dr. Blackstone take care of her."

"Do you agree with how Dr. Blackstone managed Sarah?"

"If I thought his approach were best, I would have used it."

"He disagreed with your approach, did he not?"

"He has never said as much to me."

"He changed management completely. Why?"

"That's a question for him."

"Did you tell him not to change your approach when you passed her off to him when you left?"

"I don't recall the exact conversation. That would not be my usual style, however."

"Explain."

"I usually give my reasons for doing something unusual or out of the ordinary but I don't tell people how to practice."

"You abdicated her care then?"

"Your words, not mine."

"Rather than send her to experts, you relegated her to your partner, who is not specialized in heart failure and who dislikes you, whose disdain may have carried over to his care of your patient. That seems like bad judgement to me. Was it?"

"I didn't expect him to drastically change management or to criticize me in front of the patient and her family."

"I was referring more to his expertise."

"I'll answer for my actions. He will answer for his. I had every expectation he would provide good care."

"But you think he did not do well, do you?"

"My father often quoted an old Indian adage. You should not judge a man until you have walked a mile in his moccasins. As I have said, I'm unhappy about the outcome but I was not there on the Saturday she deteriorated."

"Did you ask him why he altered your approach?"

"I don't think I did. As I recall, when he told me she died, I was too surprised to get all the details."

"So, you didn't care."

"You like putting words in my mouth."

"Dr. Harrison," Judge Bradford demanded, "I have little tolerance for nonsense."

"Mr. Ramussen is mischaracterizing my statements for the jury by the way he phrases some of his questions. What he just said wasn't a question."

She sighed loudly. "Point taken. Carry on, Counselor."

Ramussen noticed Melanie, his wife, entering the courtroom and taking a seat. He paused and refocused.

"Would you agree with me that you and Dr. Blackstone are not close friends?"

Hugh smiled. "I would."

"You have had disagreements over the years, correct?"

"Yes."

"Disagreements between you and him and other former partners led you to leave your group?"

"Yes."

"As I look at the two of you behind the defense table and at other times, I still sense conflict. Is that true?"

Judge Bradford glowered at him, wagged one finger, grasped the gavel.

"I have no idea what you sense," Harrison said.

A couple of chuckles came from the jury.

"Very clever, Doctor. I will restate. Is there conflict between you and Dr. Blackstone?"

"I have no ongoing battle with him. I think the stress of this trial has taken a toll on his patience."

"When the two of you took care of Sarah, your approaches were polar opposites, were they not?"

"They differed. Yes."

"Just as you differ on many other things, correct."

"Variety is normal. We have one jury comprised of different individuals. You and Mr.

Hart must differ as well."

"Answer the question."

"Yes."

"Prior to the incident with Sarah, you surely must have recognized that Dr. Blackstone had approaches that were quite different, did you not?"

"Yes."

"Incompatible?"

Hugh thought for a while. "That's one reason I left the Chandler Cardiovascular."

"Here's what I think, Doctor. Your dysfunctional relationship caused or at least contributed to the premature death of this young mother." A throat cleared in the back of the room, a sound Brett knew well. He didn't need to turn. But he had to swallow. He paused. "It could be that one of you was right and one of you was wrong. Were you wrong?"

"It could also be that Sarah died of a one hundred percent fatal disease and that regardless of the care she received, she was going to die."

"Is it your testimony she would've died if she had received a VAD, then a cardiac transplant?"

"No. The natural history of her disease was one hundred percent fatal. Transplant is the only option for survival. But we didn't know at that time that her disease fell into that category."

"Because you didn't send her for a biopsy at Wasatch."

"When I was taking care of her, she didn't meet criteria."

"So you say, Doctor. So you say." He turned to the jury. "For the sake of argument, let's assume that you're right. When did she meet criteria for a biopsy?"

"The day after I left."

"That would be the day your partner, one with whom you do not see eye to eye, one that doesn't share your high reputation, one that differs greatly from you, dramatically changed her treatment. Correct?"

"It was a Saturday."

"Nice dodge. But we all know what happened. No biopsy meant no diagnosis. No diagnosis led to a delay in care. A delay in care killed her. It was a delay in care that resulted in her death, was it not?"

"In part."

"Your delay?"

"I spent a week taking care of Sarah with her myocarditis, a condition that usually resolves. I was waiting for that resolution. If you think for one second that most doctors don't agonize in such situations, you are mistaken. I certainly did. At the time I spent additional time studying publications and textbooks.

"Hindsight is twenty-twenty. Now that we know she had a rare but lethal disease, it is clear I should have sent her to the Wasatch on the Friday when I left. In fact, if I knew the diagnosis from the start, I should have referred her immediately. If you know the end from the beginning, it is easy to make right decisions. But at that point it wasn't that clear."

"Do you agree that your delay in sending her for definitive care contributed to her death?"

"We pay a price when a patient dies because of something we did or didn't do, even if our decisions and actions were right. Sarah came to me in pain, with trust that I would help. I tried but as it turned out, I failed. While I think my decisions were sound, Mr. Ramussen, if the jury finds them to be malpractice, then so be it. I will not blame them, because I'm sure they, too, will do their best."

It was completely silent. Ramussen looked at Hart, who shook his head in disappointment. He walked back to his table where he and Hart whispered briefly.

Ramussen then said, "I believe I am finished with Dr. Harrison, Your Honor."

Judge Bradford looked toward the defense table. The attorneys all indicated they had no redirect questions. She directed Harrison to return to his seat. "Are you prepared for summation, Mr. Hart?"

"I need half a minute." As he shuffled quickly through several papers, Dr. Blackstone entered the court, right arm in a sling immobilizer. With a medical assistant Harrison recognized from Chandler Cardiovascular at his elbow, he waved his way unsteadily to the defense table. He paused before he sat, scowling at Doug Thompson, who flourished with one hand without returning the evil eye. They shuffled chairs, seating Blackstone against the wall, as far everyone else as possible. That put Harrison on the aisle, where the hospital attorney, Matt Parr, had been seated the whole trial.

"How are you?" Henriod whispered.

"Dislocated shoulder," he slurred. "They put it back in the socket in the ER."

Hart began his summary. "To everything there is a season and a time for every purpose under heaven. A time to be born, a time to die. A time to cast stones and a time to gather stones together. I, for one, cannot believe it was the time for Sarah Thompson to die. For those whose incompetence and lack of caring led to this terrible loss, now is the time for an accounting."

Jessop wrote furiously as he constructed his fortress of facts. Harrison took his own notes of medical misstatements and faulty conclusions.

Chapter 57

Parr, Henriod and Jessop made their concluding remarks followed by jury instructions. At 3:45 the jury left to deliberate. They agreed to stay as late as 9:00 if needed. If they could not reach a verdict by then, it would need to continue on Saturday morning. Doug Thompson ran into a pair of Salt Lake Police detectives as he exited the courtroom. They pulled him aside and slipped handcuffs on his wrists.

Thompson looked at Hart, who was nearby. "I could only get you out for the trial. Sorry."

"We don't know anything about that," one of the officers said. "You're being charged with assault, which is a violation of bail."

Harrison and Jessop walked past.

"I stopped an assault. I should get a medal, not arrested."

"We just need to take you in until we get all the facts."

"Excuse me," Hugh interjected. "I was the man Doug protected."

"We'll want to ask you questions later, sir."

"Why not right now?"

"Are you a friend of Thompson's?"

"Hardly. He is suing me for thirty million dollars."

The cop whistled. "Who are you? I thought he was suing Dr. Blackstone."

"I'm Hugh Harrison, another defendant."

"Dr. Harrison." The larger cop muttered as he wrote in a small pocket pad.

"Blackstone was punching me. Doug stopped him."

"With a punch?"

"No. He blocked one and Blackstone fell over the balustrade."

"That's a bit different than what Blackstone alleges," the cop said.

"Who has a reason to lie? He or I?"

"I don't know. You have no reason to defend this character," he said, thumb gesturing at

Doug. "In fact, you should be trashing him."

"There are other witnesses who will corroborate what I just said."

"We saw what happened."

A man stepped forward. He and his female partner were not known to Hugh. They gave their names to the police. Harrison handed his card to the officer. They removed the cuffs and let Doug go free.

Jessop led the way to the elevator, briefcase in hand, an odd smirk on her face.

"What are you thinking?" Harrison asked.

"You do the strangest things. The dirt bag who wants to ruin your life, a lifelong criminal, you defend when you don't need to. It's just crazy."

"He's an easy target. Blackstone is the problem and that loser has enough challenges without taking heat for defending me. I owe him that much."

Harrison and all the attorneys were alone in the elevator.

"I'm sure they don't want to come back on Monday, so it'll be a hasty decision, today or tomorrow," Pope speculated.

"This is going to look bad on my record," Jessop said with a grimace.

"I have more to lose that a shift in my win-loss ratio," Harrison said.

"Sorry. That was pretty insensitive. Do you want to join us for drinks, Doctor?"

They exited into the lobby.

"My phone's been buzzing for the last hour. I need to see what's up. Besides, I think I need a little time to prepare myself for the verdict."

Harrison's phone had several messages, all from Dominici. He called back expecting on the junior lawyers to answer as had happened every call in the past.

The smooth tenor answered, "Dr. Harrison, I presume."

Harrison walked slowly toward the outer doors, behind the gaggle of attorneys. "You answered your own phone. That's unusual."

"We're in Salt Lake. Spent the entire day with the justice department, the opposing counsel and a judge. I have good news and bad news."

"Not sure which I want to hear first."

"The good news is that your case hasn't been dismissed."

"That's nice."

"Auspicious proposed a settlement."

"Keep talking."

"Your group is fighting tooth and nail. No settlement from them yet. And the dollar figure is low."

"How low?"

"Less than a million."

"That sounds ridiculous."

"Indeed. So Swift, the U.S. Attorney, got tough, threatening. He gave them, both

Chandler and Auspicious, the weekend to come up with something better."

"That still good news."

"He handed them an outline of the charges he plans to file Tuesday morning, civil and criminal."

"The bad news?"

"Two senators and a slew of congressmen from California are marshaling forces to block this process. They want their cash cow to continue to squirt milk into their campaigns."

"They can do that?"

"They are involved and powerful. No telling what they can do. The judge, on the other hand, might just want to stick it to 'em, just as much as they deserve."

"This is nerve wracking."

"That's law. It's not for sissies. Anyway, Doctor, we should have another offer by the end of day Monday."

"Thanks for the call." Hugh headed for a bar on Main Street.

He ate slowly and nursed a beer until about six-thirty, when his phone rang, Jessop's number appearing on screen. "Is the verdict in?" he answered.

"And hello to you, too," she said. "Jury's headed home for the night. They'll be back for more deliberation tomorrow."

"You thought a short deliberation was not in my favor."

"Yes, so I think this is good."

"I ... I don't know what to say."

"When the jury makes a decision, we'll have around thirty minutes to appear."

"That's not a problem for me. I've go nowhere to go."

Chapter 58

Ed and Amy drove to the hospital. Myra was on the fourth floor, out of ICU and in a small private room a few doors away from where Sarah had been. She was in bed, looking as comfortable as she could, transfixed on the simple images and canned laughter emanating from the tube. She glanced at them as they entered then fumbled for the remote to decrease the sound.

"No verdict yet," Ed said.

"So, we still got no money?"

"We'll win something."

"Not thirty million?"

"I don't know. I doubt it. Plus Hart will get a third plus expenses, so a lot goes to him."

"Damn greedy lawyers!" She was getting agitated.

"I doubt either doctor has ten million in assets. At least, no one thinks so. Maybe combined they might have that much."

"They get ungodly rich off of people's pain and suffering."

"Have you considered they all might get off?"

She sat bolt upright. "Get off?" she screamed, as much as her vocal cords would allow and her face got beet red. "Scott free? They murdered our daughter!"

"The jury might agree that she had a fatal disease. Or they might give a small award so that, after Hart gets his expenses, we get zip. Even if we win a million or two, a lot of that goes to Hart and the rest goes to Amy's trust fund. Myra, you have to be realistic."

Her breathing became coarse. "If we win we could get nothing? That smelly Hart makes money and the assassins go on their merry ways? It's criminal!"

"Calm down. You just need to be prepared for bad news."

"I'll be damned! All this trouble and what for?" She could speak more than four words without a gasp. Her face began to glisten.

"It might be a lot on money, dear. And it might not. Either way, you need to relax. It'll be fine."

Amy moved away from the bed and held onto Ed. He knew he had made a mistake in the way he had tried to prepare her for reality.

"We can dream about a huge win in a trust for Amy where it will grow. We can live off my retirement and Social Security and the interest without touching the principal. We'll live high off the hog."

Myra talked over him. "Then I suppose Doug will take the whole award and we'll get noth—" Panting, she struggled to sit up.

Ed found the bed control and raised the head. She tried to talk but could not. Amy clung tighter to Ed. He hit the nurse call button.

Myra's lip tightened as she tried to exhale and started to darken. Her eyes bulged. Amy turned her face. Ed backed away.

A young waif of a nurse came in saying, "What do you need?" She needed no answer as she immediately grasped the catastrophe in progress. Her stethoscope flew off her neck and into her ears.

"Myra, what's wrong?" She listened to her lungs for a few seconds, then called out, "I need help in here!" She twisted the knob on the oxygen until the flow hissed loudly from the nasal prongs. She then ran out and quickly returned as she wheeled a portable outfit into the room. Myra's face was dark and within seconds her eyes lost focus and rolled. "Myra, stay with me. Come on."

Ed took Amy from the room as she started to shake and cry. From around the edge of the door, he watched Myra's jaw go slack. Her chest heaved, her mouth like a guppy as her efforts slowed. Two more nurses ran in and in ten seconds they paged "Code Blue" overhead. The pair walked toward the waiting area. Expansive windows looked out on a summer evening with long shadows and a cloudless sky.

Amy had never loosened her grip.

Ed was silent as he looked at the scene, remembering a wet spring afternoon when Amy's mother spiraled toward her grave, a day when he looked out on the same landscape three years earlier. He hugged her closer, her head chest high now, half a foot higher than it was then. His throat hurt deep down, the horribly familiar pain of loss. "Grandma might be going to see your mommy."

"Mommy?"

"Do you remember your mommy?"

"Picture."

His ache got worse. "Yeah. We have pictures." He moved to a row of chairs and sat after he pulled out a thin wallet. At the front was a photograph of Sarah, caught in mid laugh, eyes alive with gaiety, full of life in a perfect moment frozen in time.

"Mommy," Amy said, putting a finger on the image.

"Yes, Amy. That was your mother. She was my little girl." He blinked, his eyes becoming moist. "My little girl."

"She not little."

"She was like you once, a long time ago."

Amy was confused and returned her focus to the snapshot. "Happy," she whispered. A smile brightened her face as she rubbed the tip of her finger over Sarah's mouth.

"I hope so," Ed said. "If she's not, I...." His voice faded in thought. "Stay here, Amy. I'll be right back." She watched him hurry back into the nursing unit. He half jogged to the door of Myra's room where a small crowd had assembled. He edged inside. "Stop," he said. He repeated it louder.

All faces turned toward him.

"She doesn't want this. She just finished two weeks of life support and does not want more."

"This is her husband," her nurse said to the young woman in a white coat, a doctor who showed up in response to the code blue.

A stocky fellow was pushing on Myra's chest rhythmically bobbing up and down. An older guy in a ponytail squeezed a bag attached to the tube that had just been placed into Myra's trachea.

"It's a little late," the young physician said.

"Please," Ed said. "I should have thought to stay but I didn't."

In his mind he heard Myra nagging. *You idiot. How could you forget something so simple?*

"Please. This is cruel." He gestured at the whole circus.

"Stop," the doctor directed after considering the situation.

The chest smashing and artificial breathing ceased. One green line on the monitor changed from chaos to flat. A nurse reached up and hit the silence button to stop the screech. The room became deathly still. After half a minute, Myra heaved slightly once, her final, agonal breath. The monitor was turned off. The clinical crew moved into the hall.

Ed bowed his head and left with the others. Amy was standing at the window, looking at the green leaves and grass, the blue sky and verdant mountains, drawing figures on the glass with a greasy finger. Myra's nurse found them later, cuddled in a couch.

CHAPTER 59

Almost noon on Saturday, Harrison's phone made its annoying tune and he leapt from his desk chair, knowing immediately it was Monica Jessop. But that's not what the vaguely familiar number was. He answered.

"Hey, Hugh, this is Julie. Long time no see."

"It's been a few years."

"How are you? I heard you've had a lot of changes. And a lawsuit? You?"

"You've kept up." Harrison was confused. Julie was an old friend that he and June, when they were married, used to see frequently. The two couples traveled occasionally and had dinner frequently then. But he'd seen little of her and her husband since the divorce.

"Did you hear about June?"

"She's been trying to put me in jail for not paying enough alimony. Other than that, no."

"Really? Interesting! That could explain a few things."

"Explain what?"

"Never mind." She took a big breath. "She got married this morning."

Hugh felt a huge burden lift, closed his eyes in sweet relief.

"Hugh?"

"Really? Wow. I had no idea."

"They'd been dating for a few months. He's a bit older and well, they tied the knot."

"Were you there?"

"Yes. Her new man wanted me to let you know."

"She didn't want to do it herself."

"She didn't. I guess things are still a bit tense between you two."

"Not amicable as they say."

"He thought you'd like to know that the alimony stops."

"That's nice. Is he well off?"

"Did you think she'd marry poor? The guy's loaded, built and sold a number of tech companies."

"Good for her. She traded up."

"What's up with this lawsuit?"

"When the phone rang I thought it was my attorney calling to tell me the verdict was in."

"You're not afraid you'll lose, are you? Hard to imagine someone as good as you are would ever get sued."

"If I lose, it'll put me millions in debt. Might not be able to work and I clearly wouldn't be able to pay her alimony."

There was silence.

"That didn't have anything to do with the timing of their wedding, did it?"

"I don't know. It was short notice, though. Just a couple of days. I thought the short notice was so they could, you know, not have to put off intimacy a lot longer. So they could still qualify for a Mormon Temple wedding."

"I don't think it was sex. It was money."

"Listen to you! No wonder you two don't get along."

"You don't know her the way I do."

"No, I don't."

Early Saturday afternoon six partners of Chandler Cardiovascular and their attorney, Jon

Gullimore, met in their boardroom.

"What I'd like to know," Gullimore said, "is, how did they get this information?"

"At this point, does it matter?" Malouf asked.

"It had to be Harrison," said Monty Pierce. "I'm not sure exactly how."

"More likely it came from the files they took from your offices," Gullimore said. "Anyway, the amended complaint is pretty accurate. To defend against it, it's going to take more than me. It'll require an office full of attorneys, accountants and consultants. It'll cost somewhere far north of a million dollars."

"I thought you said everything we did was legal," Pierce said.

"We'll win," Blackstone said.

"The consent decree with Auspicious compromises the issue. We should win but that's far from certain," Gullimore said.

"Stan, if you lose your damn lawsuit," Malouf said, "we lose as well. If the award is above our coverage limits, the excess comes out of our revenue."

"Why do we lose money for his screw-up?" Ted Hatcher asked.

"Because Chandler Cardiovascular is one of the named defendants," Malouf said.

"Even if you weren't, if the award for Dr. Blackstone is beyond his ability to pay, they'll come after Chandler for the remainder," Gullimore said.

"That should fail," Pierce said.

"The way your documents read there is joint and several liability."

"Why?" Pierce asked.

"That's one way you were able to get rid of Harrison."

"He's our worst nightmare," Hatcher said amidst a chorus of murmurs and groans.

"I'm not going to lose," Blackstone said. "So, just everyone chill."

"Stan, you've settled several suits and you have three more pending," Malouf said. "You're a liability. Our malpractice premiums will increase by sixty percent next year, if you're still here. Quit, or we'll fire you."

"You can't do that!" Blackstone raised his voice.

"We have to," Pierce said. "For everyone's sake."

"I am not going to lose one single time! Not now, not ever!"

"Back on topic," Gullimore said, "you need to decide if you are willing to settle to prevent civil and criminal charges from being filed. Criminal charges mean people could go to jail. Just wanted to make that clear."

"What would a settlement look like?" Malouf said.

"Swift told me they had calculated about $2.5 million in damages at this point and they like to treble that figure. Throw in their expenses so maybe $10 million plus your own legal fees is the top number of your potential liability."

"Jon, that's ridiculous," Pierce said.

"Government extortion," Hatcher said. "We should not offer them a red cent."

"My recommendation is that we offer them a million dollars since it'll cost you at least that much to—"

"No!" Blackstone exploded. "Never! It's moral corruption. We did nothing wrong. Offer them nothing."

"We can't do that, Stan," Pierce said. "If it comes out in the papers and evening news that we have been charged with fraud, our business will take a hit."

"And there's something in there about unnecessary procedures," Malouf said. "If that gets out, we could anticipate a spate of lawsuits."

"But the settlement will make the papers," Blackstone said.

"For one day," Gullimore said, "not for weeks of a trial full of dirt."

"What if we just dissolve the entire practice?" Hatcher said.

"Won't work at this point," Gullimore said.

"What happens if Harrison goes away?" Pierce asked.

"Other than a huge celebration here?" Malouf said.

"Like if we pay him off?" Hatcher asked.

Pierce shrugged.

"He wouldn't testify," Gullimore said. "But he has made a long affidavit, which would be admissible. So the net benefit, if you paid him off, is small."

"We're giving nothing to Harrison," Blackstone said.

"That's the first thing you've said today that I agree with," Hatcher said.

"I'd rather offer to settle," Malouf said.

"I agree," Pierce said. "One million dollars."

"This is going to be a negotiation on Monday," Gullimore said. "I may need some latitude."

"You want an upper number?" Malouf asked.

"I do."

"Ten cents," Blackstone muttered.

"You're an idiot!" Pierce said. "I move that we remove Stan Blackstone from the board."

"Seconded," Obi-Poku said.

Everyone starred at him for a second, as this was so out of character. Then all talked at once. Blackstone folded his arms and stopped yelling as the torrent of discussion swirled.

Sarisha pounded on the table to get everyone to calm down. "We have a motion on the table," she spoke loudly.

"More like a movement," Blackstone said.

And the meeting went on.

In the wee hours of Sunday morning, a policeman slammed Doug against the hood of his car by a policeman. He was arrested with cocaine in his car, pockets and nose. Doug's single phone call went to Hart. He declined to get involved as he was a personal injury attorney, not criminal defense. When Hart hung up, he knew his bond money was forfeit but he would add it as an expense to the account. He no longer needed Thompson in court and his absence when the verdict was announced would be a bonus.

Harrison got the thirty-minute warning call from Jessop in mid-morning Monday. The gentle exhilaration from his alimony-free status faded as he drove in. He met the contingent of defense attorneys and Blackstone, in a sling, outside the room.

The gavel banged minutes later. Most of the jurors seemed happy.

"What say you?" Judge Bradford enunciated precisely.

"In the matter of Thompson and Szabo versus OCHA Hospital we find for the plaintiffs in the amount of $3 million."

Matt Parr looked back in fear and sympathy at Don Zone and Jennifer Hayes, who made no reaction at all.

Ed squeezed Amy's hand and she looked up at him.

"In the matter of Thompson and Szabo versus Chandler Cardiovascular we find for the plaintiffs in the amount of $5 million."

Hart leaned back with a smile, then turned to Ed and shook his hand.

"In the matter of Thompson and Szabo versus Stanton Blackstone, we find for the plaintiffs in the amount of $10 million."

This was followed by gasps in the gallery.

Blackstone's jaw dropped in disbelief. His eyes widened as he stared at the jury. Zone and Hayes looked at each other with incredulity. Behind them, Montgomery Pierce groaned audibly. Malouf's head went back, her eyes to the ceiling.

Harrison bowed his head and stretched his neck, waiting for the execution.

"In the matter of Thompson and Szabo versus Hugh H. Harrison, we find for the defendant."

Hart jerked then looked at Ramussen. He shrugged.

In the stunning silence a hundred eyes focused on Harrison, whose mouth gaped as he looked at the jury foreman who smiled back. Jessop hugged him, shook him and beamed with the brightest smile he had ever seen.

"I object to the award, Your Honor," Henriod said.

"Your objection is noted," she replied, then faced the jury. "Thank you for your service. This matter is concluded."

The gavel ended Harrison's part of the three-year nightmare with a slap. He collapsed, blinking, seeing nothing, stunned.

"Thank you, Mr. Hart. You did a great job." Ed shook his hand. "I think the jury got it right."

"Not sure it was totally correct but we have an $18 million award, a huge award," Hart said, seeing a net of over five million dollars in his bank account. "Your granddaughter will have money for her care if you manage it right. I can give you some guidance about that when the time comes."

"It was the best outcome, better than I had hoped," Ramussen said.

"I think your gaffe got Harrison off," Hart said.

"I hope so," he replied.

"I agree," Ed said. "I think he got tarred by his loser partner."

"Now we'll probably need to get through the objection to omitting the damages phase," Hart said. "Getting all of the money will be harder because Dr. Blackstone's insurance limit is one million. He'll need to liquidate assets including his home and retirement. We'll garnish his wages to pay the rest. That will be a slower process. And we can go after his group's income to make up the deficit. It'll be like a ten-year-long root canal for them all." Hart rubbed his hands and smiled. "This should make your wife happy."

Ed said nothing in response.

"You're still the legal guardian, right?" Ramussen asked.

Ed nodded.

"It'll be permanent, I suspect," Hart said. "Thompson's back in jail. Arrested yesterday. He shouldn't be getting out for a long time, well after Amy is an adult."

Ed smiled.

Harrison sat numbly in the wooden chair, mentally paralyzed.

Jessop placed a hand on his shoulder. "Congratulations, Doc. I don't know exactly how we did it but it's done."

"Ah," Hugh cleared his throat as he tried to find his voice. "Thank you," he finally said. "I can't believe it."

She smiled again both in pride.

Franklin Pope approached. He bent his six-and-a-half-foot frame down and hugged attorney Jessop enthusiastically. She lacked a similar response.

"Great job," he said, then let go. "You saved us a million bucks. I'm speechless. I'm shocked. I'm—"

"I really have no idea how that happened," she said. "The jury laid it all on Blackstone. All of it. The hospital and the practice were just collateral damage."

"Congratulations, Doctor." Frank held a hand down to Hugh, who was still seated.

Hugh shook it. "I'm speechless."

"You're a very good physician. Don't let this discourage you."

"I was lucky. And well represented. I guess you had a win and a loss."

"Well, we lost one million instead of two. Not exactly a win but I'm grateful for it. Jessop did a great job." He clapped her on the shoulder again.

Simultaneously at the other end of the defense table, Blackstone's head was face down covered by his one good arm, mumbling. Henriod left him alone and scanned the crowd, expecting to see Stacey Blackstone. She had never appeared.

Blackstone stood abruptly. "This is wrong," he said to no one. "Someone must have tampered with the jury."

"We'll appeal, Dr. Blackstone," Henriod said. "I'll start this afternoon."

"There must have been something illegal here. I could not have lost this case without somebody monkeying around behind the scenes."

Pope moved from Harrison to Blackstone. "Doctor, you did what you could," he said.

"I'm not sure how the verdict ended up so screwy." He then shook Henriod's hand. "I'm sorry."

"Somebody is going to be sorry," Blackstone said. His nostrils flared. "If Harrison had anything to do with this, and it looks that way to me, I'll make him regret he was ever born."

"He had no way of influencing the result outside of what he did in the courtroom," Pope said.

"You have no idea what he is capable of doing. He is devious and a profligate manipulator, evil to the core."

"I understand your anger," Henriod began, but Blackstone pushed past him, shaking his left forefinger, since his right was in a sling, at Harrison.

"I don't know how you won, Hugh, but I'll find out."

Pope and Henriod restrained Blackstone.

"I'll make you regret the day you were born."

"Sorry you lost."

"You son of a bitch. I'll destroy you. I'll kill you."

"Enough!" Pope said. "Get a hold of yourself."

"This is not Dr. Harrison's fault," Henriod said. "And never threaten to kill anyone, especially in a court of law, you—" He swallowed his epithet.

"This shall not stand," Blackstone said. "God will prevail."

"I hope she does," Hugh said, as he had so many times before, just to irritate him. "Augh!" Blackstone screamed and lunged at Harrison.

He walked out of the room as two attorneys and a bailiff restrained his former partner.

CHAPTER 59

Gullimore waited in the conference room until Pierce and Malouf returned from court.

"I heard you were at the malpractice verdict. How'd that go?"

"It was bad," Malouf said. "Our group got hit with a five-million-dollar award. Blackstone lost $10 million."

"That's awful. Huge! Whoa, that's really bad."

One of the office secretaries was in the room, getting other members of the Chandler board on a conference call. "But, it'll get worse."

"Don't get Blackstone on the call," Pierce directed the secretary.

It was not long before Pierce, Hatcher, and Obi-Poku joined the call.

Gullimore spoke. "I had to offer two-point-five million to settle. I know that's more than

I was authorized but Swift was adamant that the government be made whole by the amount."

"We don't have anywhere near that amount," Malouf said.

"Is your offer final? Like in writing?" Pierce asked.

"I have an hour to get it approved by you. Fifty minutes at this point."

"Don't do it," Malouf said. "Guys, you may not know it yet but Blackstone lost his case.

$10 million from him and $5 million from us. Our insurance will cover one million, so $4 million comes from our revenue."

"You'll appeal, right?" Gullimore asked, after a burst of profanities subsided.

"Of course," Malouf said. "But still, I can't see offering a settlement of $2.5 million after we just lost 5."

"Five million here, two million there and pretty soon you're talking about real money,"

Hatcher said.

"Not funny," Pierce said

"I think you need to approve this settlement," Gullimore said. "It's more likely than not that you'll lose if you go to court. Auspicious is likely to settle and if they admit culpability, they could reduce the fine. That admission be admissible in your trial, if it gets that far. I'm afraid this is your only reasonable option."

"Why would they settle?" Pierce asked.

"Their behavior was a direct violation of a consent decree from a few years earlier. If they don't settle they could lose over a billion dollars."

"What does a whistleblower get?" Pierce asked.

"Maybe five to fifteen percent."

"Holy shit!" came from three of the voices on the call.

"We should settle, Sarisha," Pierce said. "Then we dissolve or declare bankruptcy."

"The joint and several liability will follow all stockholders wherever you go," Gullimore said. "But, as terrible as it is and despite the abysmal timing, this is the best deal you'll get.

And no one admits guilt or goes to jail. Which means you all keep your license to practice."

For a moment no one spoke.

"I don't want to go to jail," Hatcher said.

"I move we settle," Pierce said. "It's the least bad option."

All the male voices agreed.

"Okay," Sarisha said. "Jon, make it happen."

"One more thing," Pierce said. "How do we get rid of Blackstone? Doesn't costing the practice $5 million some sort of breach of contract, a *for-cause* termination event?"

"It is," Gullimore said.

"I move we fire his ass," Pierce said.

The vote was instantaneous and unanimous in affirmation.

Five days after the trial ended Harrison waited near noon in front of the Samaritan hospital. Jana hurried out wearing black jeans and a pale silk blouse and climbed in the car.

"I'm sorry. Did you wait long?"

"Less than a minute."

She settled into the seat, clicking her belt, adjusting her hair and clothing. Her eyes rested on Hugh as he exited into traffic.

"It's good to see you in the middle of the day," she said.

"It's nice to see you anytime," he countered happily.

She gave her signature chuckle, a single, short exhale out her nose with a barely audible hmmm, the pitch shaped like a comma. He loved to hear it.

After a short drive they entered a drive and passed under a wrought-iron arch. Sunset Lawn, a mortuary sprawled out in resplendent grass and a variety of trees. One of three small signs said "Szabo" and pointed left.

"None of the docs can stop talking about your trial. It has been the hot topic. It has them scared witless."

"It was a massive award, frightening."

"They have given you god-status, like you won the World Series or the Super Bowl." "That's a little lame, don't you think?"

"Of course not. I think you're great. Why shouldn't they? Besides, it destroys Chandler and hurts OCHA, which they like."

The car slowed as they approached a small group of vehicles pulled to the side and a group of people loitering. Harrison parked. As they neared the small crowd, eight men stood behind a hearse and caught the heavy casket as it rolled out. Struggling, they made their way to the gravesite, onto Astroturf and then positioned Myra's unwieldy remains onto the straps that would lower her into the ground. Four wreaths stood on metal stands and several other sprays of flowers surrounded the area, adding a funereal fragrance to the almost still-warm air.

"Thanks for coming with me," Harrison said.

"I'm sure you'll pay me back," she responded.

They held at the outskirts, watching.

Amy stayed at Ed's side. Ed looked good, lighter in gait, shaking hands, hugging back when needed. Harrison looked for Doug Thompson without result.

A black-suited man, almost certainly a funeral director, said a few sentences to the group and backed away. A tall, large man came to the foot of the casket, cleared his throat and began to speak.

"That's my older sister lying there in peace." He gestured and sniffed his tears back up his nose. "We all know this day will come for each of us, but you're never truly ready."

The sun was hot. Harrison unfolded an umbrella and put it above Jana and him. He put an arm around Jana, who returned the gesture. He watched Amy, who in turn watched others in the family gathered near. A couple of vignettes from childhood and a list of positive traits passed through the atmosphere and the little brother stopped speaking.

"I thought about burying Myra in her recliner," Ed said. "But the city ordinances insist on a hermetically sealed casket."

There was polite laughter. Ed wore a hat that was vaguely in style but also could have come from the prohibition era, keeping his face in shadow.

"She has her favorite quilt in the casket with her, one that she and Sarah made about twenty years ago. They liked to quilt. Women talk while they sew. It's a good way to build relationships. They may be talking now, once again, the first time in over three years." Ed did not cry. His voiced wavered sometimes but never faltered.

"Myra was a real knock-out when I married her. But, life takes a toll." He lofted his hat and mopped his head with a handkerchief quickly. Ed stepped away from the speaking place, bent down and hugged Amy.

A pastor came forward and began speaking about life after death, inevitable from a cleric. Harrison recalled that, historically, the resurrection notion began with Greek mythology where life sprang from death often, like the children Cronus ate then vomited up as living adults years later.

Afterward, Ed came over to them. "Thank you for coming."

"I'm sorry for your loss," Harrison said. "Thanks for letting me know. I didn't think you would like me here."

"Not at all. It was your partner that misled us about you. Then Myra and Doug wouldn't let it go. Hart was all about the money. What a debacle."

Amy held on to Ed's arm, looking away.

"This is my friend, Jana."

She extended her hand. Ed took it and shook it gently.

"You'll have resources to take care of Amy for the rest of her life."

"If we survive the appeals. If we can collect the money. If I can keep the money away from Doug. But it looks like I'll get complete legal guardianship and cut him completely out. None of this is certain."

"Nothing is."

"Except death," he said.

"I wish you well, Ed."

"Likewise," he said.

When they drove away, they saw Amy still attached to Ed's side.

"I think Ed and Myra had a difficult relationship. I think she treated him like a slave."

"He probably enabled her behavior and got what he created," Jana said.

"Oh. And when did you go so objective?"

"I'm just saying what you would. It's logical, unemotional, factual, a dose of your own medicine."

"Using my own methods to bring me back to reality?"

"You are rubbing off on me."

"Rubbing can be so much fun."

"Too bad you're working in Oregon and Texas and South Dakota. We'll have little opportunity to hang out."

"Guy's gotta make a living."

"Can't you work in town? I bet someone at Good Sam would hire you. You're a rock star."

"I tried. I'm radioactive. This is the only gig I can get."

"That was before you avoided losing that lawsuit."

"Failing to lose is not the same as winning."

"You can be a butthead, you know."

"I always thought I was just a nice guy."

"Ha!"

Chapter 60

A dry two-lane highway sped beneath Blackstone's black Infinity in the early morning blackness. A stack of letters rested on the passenger seat, worn and wrinkled from repeated reading. One was from the malpractice insurance company notifying him that he was no longer insurable. On top of that was a letter obviously written by Jonathan Gullimore, the attorney for Chandler Cardiovascular. It was on the CCC letterhead and over the signatures of his three now former partners who governed the practice as the trilogy: Richard Black, Montgomery Pierce and Chimwuanya Obi-Poku. It informed him of his termination for cause. Under those were a couple of notices that he had been terminated from hospital staffs and his privileges revoked. All were dated months earlier.

An eleven-by-fourteen-inch photograph sat atop the letters, taken two years earlier in happier days. He and Stacey smiled, as did Rachel. Now he was functionally single and broke. His wife and child had returned to Oklahoma. His home had been sold, his possessions liquidated, his wages, while he had any, garnished.

Curse God and die.

Stacey had been arrested for moving a large amount of money out of the country. Once it had been returned and given to the trust fund for Amy Thompson she was released with a guilty plea. Now she worked at a packing plant for a decent wage but a huge decrease in her standard of living. Rachel was in Kindergarten for half the day and in day care the rest of the time.

Blackstone engaged in hours of prayer, sometimes in his apartment and other times deep in the desert where he could raise his voice like prophets of old, calling loudly on God.

"Oh, God, why have all the things I cherish been swept away? Am I as Job? I have obeyed thy word, kept myself clean from the corruption of the world. My abusers prosper and I am in the depths of despair. Oh, God, please bring an end to my punishment. Make known to me why thou dost seek to humble me so."

He took another gulp from his Jose Cuervo Tequila. Desert sped past.

"Please, oh, God Almighty, work a change in the heart of my Stacey that she will honor and obey her husband. Let her see I did no wrong. Let my precious daughter remember me with fondness and love me with the guileless, unconditional love of the young.

"That the reward of my intellect and skill go to Ed Szabo is more than I can bear. Smite him and his cursed grandchild so that this heavy load can be lifted. Let the breath of thy potent lips sweep away the many others who persecute me in order to line their pockets with the fruits of my honest labor. Why dost thou permit this evil, oh, God?"

Swerving in the black ribbon highway cut in the red rock desert of southern Utah he took another swallow. The two-quart bottle, fresh from the liquor store the previous evening was more than three quarters empty. Smooth and tasty at first, he did not drink it now to enjoyment. He capped the bottle and put it back on the floor, swerving in the cold January air. The snow covered Sierra LaSalle peaks in Colorado to the east glowed in the light of the full moon, beautiful and majestic. Patches of snow dotted the high desert, flashing past the windows. The road was dry.

Blackstone pounded the steering wheel with his fists and screamed at the top of lungs, his voice now hoarse, cursing Jesus, Stacey, Malouf, Harrison, God, Pierce and a long list of others that had contributed to his agony. "Art thou deaf, God?" he bellowed.

He heard a voice. "Not yet."

He gripped tightly and looked around, in the back seat, outside the windows. He corrected hard and fishtailed briefly to avoid going off the road. "I was not seeking a sign. Just a reply of the most subtle variety. But I just heard thy voice."

"Trust in God especially when it seems he has deserted you."

"Why hast thou deserted me?"

"Some days it rains on the just and the unjust."

"I love you, God."

"Show me."

"How?"

"Take the next turn, the dirt road just ahead."

"This is how I show my love?"

"Have a little faith."

The tires screeched as he braked to make the turn onto a dirt road. The car bounced and creaked as it went along.

"This looks promising," the voice said.

"The road is getting pretty bad."

"Take a drink. It'll steady your nerves."

Stan took several swallows, bringing tears to his eyes. He took a few more and dropped the almost empty bottle onto the floor.

"Now, put the pedal to metal. It'll be fun. I will catch you and bring you to safety."

"Honest?"

"I'll give you proof, eighty proof that I exist."

"It'll be fun?"

"Faster, Stan, down the straight and narrow."

Blackstone accelerated, tires spitting gravel as his speed increased. As he neared a curve, he had a loss of faith. He slammed on the brakes and turned the wheel. The road disappeared.

He was weightless when her heard the voice again, "Oh, ye of little faith." Blackstone's scream ended abruptly.

Chapter 61

Three days later, Hugh stopped on Norm's Island in the Yellowstone River, breath hanging in the air in the January cold. He was jogging in Riverfront Park, a few minutes from his hotel. It was about twenty minutes back to his car, as far away as he dared go while on cardiology call for the emergency room of Saint Vincent's Hospital. The river flowed mostly under thick, static ice. Where the current was stronger, a narrow slit of water was visible. The geese were gone in mid-winter. The sun at noon hung low in the south and today gave a vague hint of its location through high clouds moving quickly southeast. He panted, lungs burning from frigid exposure. The high of day, in a few hours was predicted to be two degrees.

The snow was only ankle deep off the path where dogs and their walkers tramped it into ice. It was his long lunch break, allowed because his work was done and no one cared if he was on site, just able to respond within half an hour. He had worked in Missoula, Helena, Kalispell and Great Falls, all the big towns of Montana. Billings was the biggest of them all with a burgeoning one hundred ten thousand people. He was one of very few interventional cardiologists with a license to practice in Montana, so he was in great demand.

Heading back to his car through the snow and fallen leaves his phone jangled. He had to take his glove off, reach deep inside a pocket and pull it out, a clumsy and long process. The number with an area code of 310 was vaguely familiar.

"Harrison," he answered.

"Where do you want me to wire your money?"

"Who is this?"

"Melissa from Higgins Cowen. We have received some of the settlement."

"That was quick."

"Funny. It's never fast. A year and a half isn't a big surprise for an amount this big. Where are you?"

"Billings, Montana."

"Skiing any good?"

"Too flat around here for downhill."

"Can you give me a routing number and an account number so I can get this money to you tomorrow?"

"Send me an email and I'll reply with the numbers when I get back to my hotel."

"Will do."

There was a lull.

"Anything else?" Hugh asked.

"Aren't you curious about the amount?"

"I'm too cold to think."

"Around forty million."

"Taxes will take half of that."

"You poor guy."

"You guys must have come out pretty well, too." His phone chimed with an incoming call.

"Thanks to you."

"I've got to answer another call. Email me."

He switched to the other call. "Forty-seven-year-old woman with chest pain," the ER doc said. "Her ECG is not bad but her pain is."

"I'll be there in twenty minutes." Harrison jogged through the snow to his car a mile away.

Eighty minutes after he arrived, he was showing the patient and her fifteen-year-old boy the angiogram pictures in the cath lab suite, explaining that an artery had been occluded but now was open. Her prospects looked good, the crisis was averted. She would be home soon within a couple of days with luck. She reached up with both hands wanting to shake his hand. He extended it.

"Thank you, thank you. You saved my life." A single tear slid down her cheek.

"I'm so glad you were here," the son said. "That was fast."

"You're welcome. That's what I do." Hugh was again embarrassed by the effusive gratitude.

After the paperwork and dictation, after finishing a short stack of echocardiograms and ECGs, he drove to the hotel in the dark. A few minutes after he entered his empty room his phone buzzed. Jana's name glowed from the screen.

"Hi, sweetie," he answered.

"How was your day?"

"Higgins Cowen called. Some money is headed our way."

"I'd be happier if you were headed my way."

"It's a lot of money."

"Money doesn't hug. It makes no dorky puns, has no wit or insight, and doesn't bring me Irish cream coffee on lazy Sunday mornings."

He smiled and wanted to come home a few days early.

www.ingramcontent.com/pod-product-compliance
Lightning Source LLC
Chambersburg PA
CBHW061504180526
45171CB00001B/27